OFF TO A GOOD START

Social and Emotional Development of Memphis Children

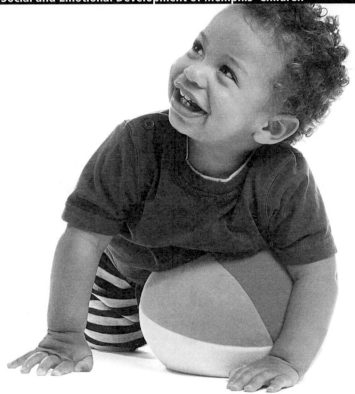

THE
URBAN
CHILD
INSTITUTE ®

RAND
CORPORATION

Library of Congress Cataloging-in-Publication Data is available for this publication

ISBN: 978-0-8330-8846-8

Published by The Urban Child Institute, Memphis, Tenn.

and

the RAND Corporation, Santa Monica, Calif.

© Copyright 2014 The Urban Child Institute and RAND Corporation

The Urban Child Institute

The Urban Child Institute (UCI) is a non-profit organization dedicated to the wellbeing and health of children from conception to three years old in Memphis and Shelby County. UCI is a data-driven, result-oriented coalition of researchers, strategists, practitioners, parents, and community members dedicated to turning knowledge and research into measurable change.

The Urban Child Institute is working to become a recognized leader in child advocacy research, a trustworthy community partner, and a place of choice for expertise, advice, and collaboration for those who want to improve the lives of children in Shelby County, Tennessee.

www.urbanchildinstitute.org

The RAND Corporation

The RAND Corporation is a research organization that develops solutions to public policy challenges to help make communities throughout the world safer and more secure, healthier and more prosperous. RAND is nonprofit, nonpartisan, and committed to the public interest.

RAND's publications do not necessarily reflect the opinions of its research clients and sponsors.

RAND® is a registered trademark.

www.rand.org

INTRODUCTION

The Urban Child Institute (UCI) began publication of the *Data Book: The State of Children in Memphis and Shelby County* in 2006 to inspire action by encouraging data-driven decisions, illuminating the challenges and opportunities facing our community, and shaping a community-wide conversation about the importance of ensuring every child a fair start in life.

Since that time, the community has frequently used the annual Data Book, citing statistics from it in local discussions, policy development, and grant applications. UCI also invested in a longitudinal study of 1,500 Shelby County mother-child dyads, known as CANDLE, that uniquely brings together biological, physical, and behavioral data to further our understanding of the drivers of early child well-being.

This year, UCI took a step back and asked ourselves how children in Shelby County are doing and where we, as a community, still have challenges. It was important to conduct this examination to ensure the Data Book was useful to the community and to identify how the Data Book can uniquely contribute to local work. Our analysis was clear—unless our children have the supports and nurturing environments to thrive, their future and the future of our community will not be bright. While UCI spent many years focusing on cognitive outcomes and the science of brain development, other important issues—like the social and emotional well-being of our children—deserved more attention.

But why social and emotional development and why now? In order for children to flourish and succeed in the 21st century, they must be able to problem solve, to develop resilience and handle stress, and to interact appropriately with peers and adults. But these abilities are not acquired overnight; brain science demonstrates that the foundation for these skills is laid early. While there is significant national focus on the racial/ethnic and economic disparities in academic achievement and other cognitive outcomes, far less attention has been paid to the capacities that help build social and emotional skills. Unfortunately, our community faces all the stressors that can impede child social and emotional growth. We have difficult community conditions, such as violence and poverty. However, we also have the assets that support healthy social and emotional development, such as a strong faith and nonprofit community. Through this book, UCI calls for a dialogue on how to support the youngest members of our community and catalyze action in this direction.

What is new? You may notice a few differences in the 2014 Data Book, now called *Off to a Good Start: Social and Emotional Development of Memphis' Children*. First, we organize our discussion around themes related to child social and emotional development, whereas the original Data Book series focused on cognitive development and the science of the brain. We hope that by organizing the book in this way, diverse community stakeholders (nonprofits, health professionals, faith community leaders, educational and human services, providers, parents, and policymakers) can use the book in different ways. Readers can still draw out data specifically relevant to their concerns and interests. But it is also possible to read individual sections one at a time, or read the whole book cover to cover to obtain the full story of children in Shelby County. Second, we have created more sections in each chapter. We include an explanation of why the topic matters, summary data from local and national sources, and recommendations for community action. In adding this detail, we hope the book grounds the discussion more firmly in scientific evidence. Finally, we have partnered with the RAND Corporation, a leading nonprofit research and policy analysis organization, which helped UCI reconceptualize the purpose, content, and rigor of the evidence summarized in *Off to a Good Start*.

Off to a Good Start is simply one part of The Urban Child Institute's vision for the future. We hope you will enjoy the new look and orientation of this year's book. We encourage your comments and your stories of how you use *Off to a Good Start* in your efforts on behalf of Shelby County children.

Eugene K. Cashman Jr.

President & CEO

The Urban Child Institute

ACKNOWLEDGMENTS

The Urban Child Institute's *Off to a Good Start: Social and Emotional Development of Memphis' Children* could not be produced and distributed without the help of numerous people.

The publication was written and produced under the general direction of Laurie Martin, Sc.D., MPH, and Lisa Sontag-Padilla, Ph.D., at the RAND Corporation. The RAND Corporation is a nonprofit institution that helps improve policy and decisionmaking through research and analysis. For more information about RAND, please visit http://www.rand.org.

Additionally, Jill Cannon, Ph.D., Anita Chandra, Dr.P.H., Anamarie Auger, Ph.D., Courtney Kase, MPH, Ryan Kandrack, B.S., and Teague Ruder, M.A., from the RAND Corporation and Catherine Joyce, M.A., Rebecca Diamond, B.A., and Katherine L. Spurlock, MSSW, MBA, from The Urban Child Institute served as contributing authors for the book. The RAND team provided the conceptual framework and analytic capacity for *Off to a Good Start,* while the UCI team offered important local context and additional data detail. Finally, special thanks are also due to Dori Walker from the RAND Corporation for design and layout.

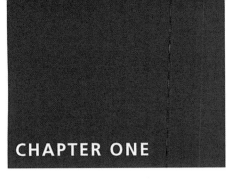

CHAPTER ONE

WHAT DO WE KNOW ABOUT
Social and Emotional Development in Early Childhood?

The first years last a lifetime.

Children's experiences in their earliest years affect how their brains work, the way they respond to stress, and their ability to form trusting relationships. During these years the brain undergoes its most dramatic growth, setting the stage for social and emotional development. Language blossoms, basic motor abilities form, thinking becomes more complex, and children begin to understand their own feelings and those of others.

From the first day of life to the first day of school, a child grows at a phenomenal pace.

Did you know?

- A child's brain doubles in size in the first year, and by age three it reaches 80 percent of its adult volume [1, 2].

- The back-and-forth interactions of babies and adults shape a baby's brain architecture, supporting the development of communication and social skills [3, 4].

- What happens in the first years of life is directly related to children's long-term cognitive, emotional, and social outcomes through adulthood [3, 4].

Want to know more?

To learn more about the importance of the first three years of life, go to

http://www.urbanchildinstitute.org/firstyears

http://www.urbanchildinstitute.org/why-0-3

http://www.urbanchildinstitute.org/articles/perceptions/soft-skills-and-success-go-hand-in-hand

All aspects of child development are interconnected **(Figure 1.1)**. For example, a child's ability to learn new information is influenced by his ability to interact appropriately with others and his ability to control his immediate impulses.

FIGURE 1.1

THINKING ABOUT THE WHOLE CHILD

Domains of development

Emotional, cognitive, social, and physical development are interrelated and influence each other.

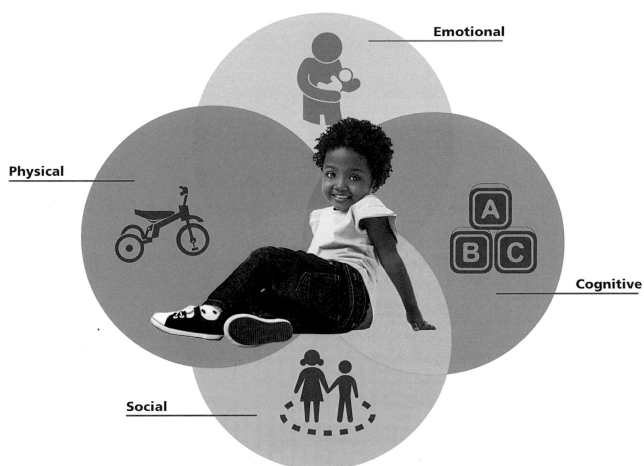

Emotional

Physical

Cognitive

Social

What is the CANDLE Study?

In 2006, The Urban Child Institute and the University of Tennessee Department of Preventative Medicine started a large-scale study of 1,500 pregnant women, starting in their second trimester, to identify what factors during pregnancy and early childhood affect a child's development and ability to learn. The CANDLE (Conditions Affecting Neurocognitive Development and Learning in Early Childhood) team recruited women ages 16–40 who were between 16 and 28 weeks pregnant to participate, drawing from Regional One Health, other community clinics, and the general community. Women had generally healthy pregnancies and, similar to Shelby County mothers who recently gave birth, were mostly African-American and low-income women. The CANDLE study follows these women and their children until the child's fifth birthday.

Want to know more?

To learn more about the CANDLE study, go to http://candlestudy.com

In Shelby County, the CANDLE Study has collected biological, physical, and behavioral data to help us better understand these connections and their collective influence on child well-being.

What is social and emotional development?

Social and emotional development is the change over time in children's ability to react to and interact with their social environment. Social and emotional development is complex and includes many different areas of growth. Each is described in more detail below:

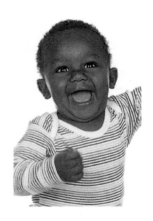

- **temperament:** the way a young child acts and responds to different situations, caregivers, and strangers

- **attachment:** the emotional bond between a child and caregiver

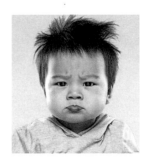

- **social skills or social competence:** the ability to get along with other people

- **emotion regulation:** the ability of a child to control his or her emotions and reactions to the environment.

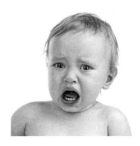

FIGURE 1.2

MILESTONES OF SOCIAL AND EMOTIONAL DEVELOPMENT

from birth through four years old

 BIRTH TO 3 MONTHS

From the start, babies eagerly explore their world, including themselves and other people. They can:

 3 TO 6 MONTHS

Babies are more likely to initiate social interaction. They begin to:

 6 TO 9 MONTHS

Babies show a wider emotional range and stronger preferences for familiar people. Most can:

 Imitation and self-regulation ga importance. Most can:

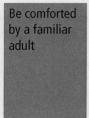 Be comforted by a familiar adult

Smile and show pleasure in response to social interaction

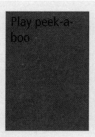 Play peek-a-boo

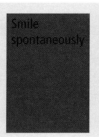 Smile spontaneously

Express several clearly differentiated emotions

Distinguish friends from strangers

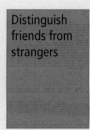 Mimic simple actions

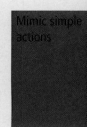

SOURCE: Adapted from http://www.pbs.org/wholechild/abc/social.html

Figure 1.2 provides examples of key social and emotional milestones for young children. Children develop in all of these areas of growth from birth through four years. These milestones help us know whether children are developing "on time." They also help us know what to expect children to understand and do at certain ages.

Question:

What should parents do if they are concerned about their child's development?

Answer:

Social and emotional milestones let us know if a child is gaining skills in the time frame we would expect. However, sometimes children will be a bit early or a bit late on some of these milestones. If parents have concerns about their child's development, encourage them to speak to their pediatrician.

Want to know more?

For a full list of milestones, go to

http://www.pbs.org/wholechild/abc/social.html

What is temperament?

Have you ever noticed how babies have personalities, even from the day they are born? Temperament is the beginning of personality. It typically refers to the way a young child acts and responds to different situations, and how he or she interacts with caregivers and strangers. Most children fall into one of three temperament categories: easy, slow-to-warm-up, and difficult [5].

**TO 12
MONTHS**

 **1 YEAR
TO 2 YEARS**

**Children become more aware
of themselves and their ability
to make things happen. At this
stage, most can:**

 **2 YEARS
TO 3 YEARS**

**Children begin to explore
everything, showing a stronger
sense of self and expanded
range of self-help skills. They
begin to:**

 **3 YEARS
TO 4 YEARS**

**Children become
more interested
in other children.
They are more
likely to:**

Show anxiety when separated from primary caregiver

Show pride and pleasure at new accomplishments

Show a strong sense of self through assertiveness, directing others to do things

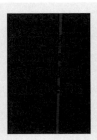

Initiate or join in play with other children

Share toys

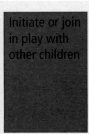

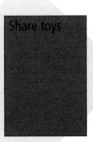

- **Easy babies,** for example, have regular sleeping times, are easily soothed when upset and are generally positive.
- **Slow-to-warm-up babies** are more hesitant in new situations and with unfamiliar people.
- **Difficult babies** are easily agitated and very sensitive to all sights and sounds.

Given that children have different temperaments, parents and other caregivers need to learn how to create environments that best support their children's temperaments [6].

DATA FACT:

- Nationally, more than half (55 percent) of infants display at least one characteristic of a difficult temperament most of the time, suggesting that many of these characteristics are common **(Figure 1.3)**. For instance, most infants want attention and company. However, when an infant demands attention through crying, fits, or whimpering most of the time, this may be a sign of a difficult temperament. And, together these behaviors make caring for difficult babies challenging for many parents. In fact, 22 percent of infants displayed two or more of these characteristics most of the time.

- SOURCE: Early Childhood Longitudinal Study, Birth Cohort (ECLS-B), 9-month data wave (2001–2002), parent report of child displaying characteristic "most times."

Question:

What does a child who is slow-to-warm-up or difficult need?

Answer:

Keep the home and outside environment as predictable as possible. At the same time, gently expose the child to new experiences. This may help foster the child's social and emotional development in a way that supports the child's unique needs.

FIGURE 1.3

SIGNS OF DIFFICULT TEMPERAMENT

Percent of infants who display behavior **most times**

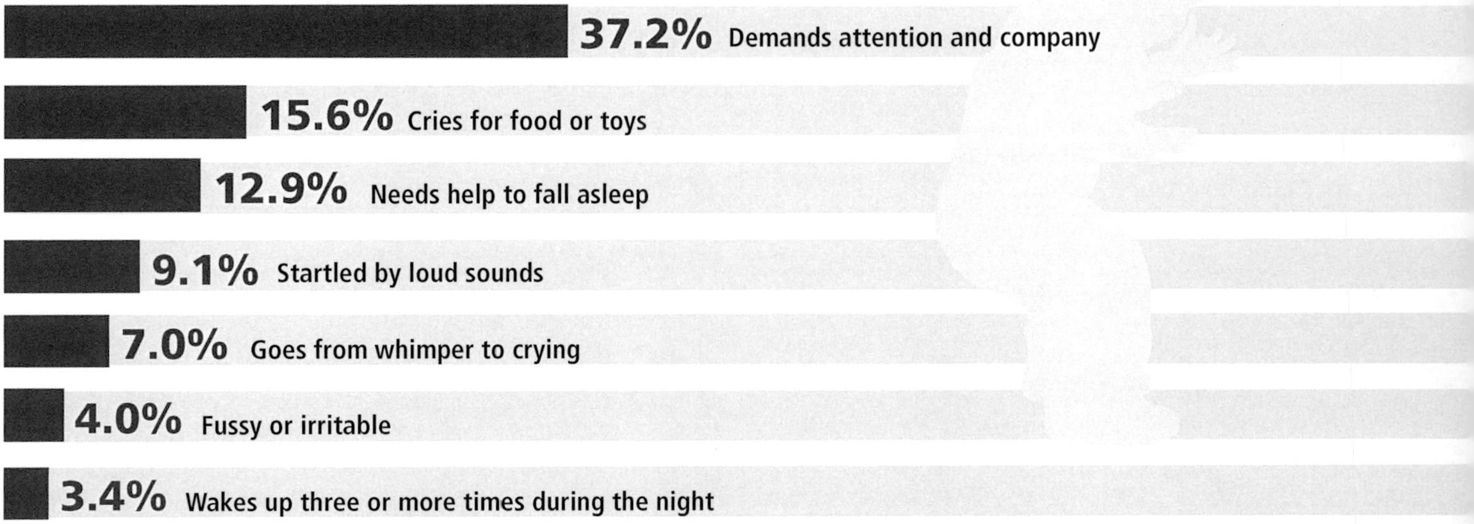

37.2% Demands attention and company

15.6% Cries for food or toys

12.9% Needs help to fall asleep

9.1% Startled by loud sounds

7.0% Goes from whimper to crying

4.0% Fussy or irritable

3.4% Wakes up three or more times during the night

SOURCE: Early Childhood Longitudinal Study, Birth Cohort (ECLS-B), 9-month data wave (2001-2002), parent report of child displaying characteristic "most times"

What is attachment?

Attachment is the emotional bond between a child and caregiver [7, 8]. The ability to form an attachment is present from birth and plays two important roles for young children. First, it motivates children to stay near a caregiver, which keeps them safe. Second, it allows children to depend on their caregiver as a source of support as they explore their surroundings. Children who do this successfully have what is often called "secure attachment."

The development of a secure attachment is important for many reasons:

- **Promotes** a positive relationship between a child and caregiver

- **Decreases** risk for social and emotional problems later in childhood and adulthood

- **Encourages** healthy relationships outside the home (e.g., child-care providers, friends, other adults)

- **Fosters** positive, trusting relationships in middle childhood, adolescence, and adulthood. [9, 10].

DATA FACT:

- Nationally, about two-thirds (62–66 percent) of infants and toddlers have secure attachment styles [7, 8].

Source: NICHD Study of Early Child Care and Youth Development: Phase I, 1991-1995

What is social competence?

Social competence refers to a person's ability to get along with others and adapt to new situations [11]. Children learn social skills very early in life that determine their social competence. For example, babies make eye contact, imitate facial expressions, and respond to voices. As children age, they interact more with other children and adults, which helps them to learn additional social skills.

Nationally, the percentage of high-risk infants in the Early Head Start Family and Child Experiences Survey (Baby FACES) that are socially competent at age one is 90 percent [12]. Using the same measure, in Shelby County, more than three-quarters (78 percent) of children age 12 months participating in the CANDLE study are considered socially competent by a parent.

SOURCE: CANDLE Study (2009–2012) Parent report of social competence measured by the Brief Infant Toddler Social Emotional Assessment (BITSEA)

Did you know?

▪ Play gives children a chance to practice different social skills. They learn to acknowledge others' feelings, play "nicely," share, and resolve conflict.

▪ As children get older, play becomes more interactive, further improving their social skills and preparing them for more active social interactions inside and outside the home.

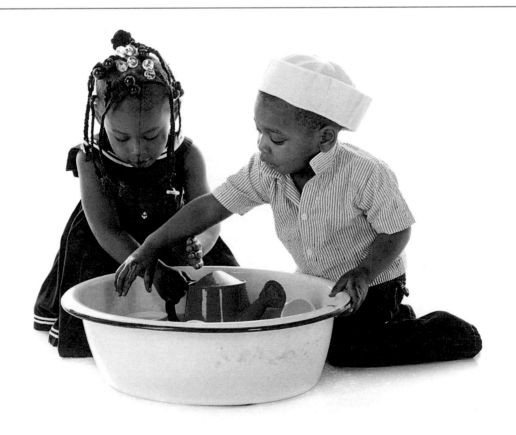

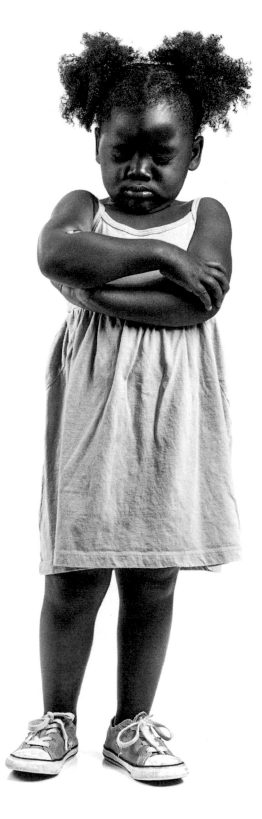

What is emotion regulation?

Emotion regulation is the ability of a child to control his or her emotions and reactions to his or her environment. This does not mean that a child should be happy, brave, and calm all of the time. It is normal, for example, for babies to cry to communicate needs or for toddlers to throw temper tantrums and push boundaries. But some children have a harder time calming down.

DATA FACT:

- Nationally, approximately 26 percent of children 12 months of age exhibited problem behaviors related to a lack of emotion regulation [12]. Using the same measure, approximately 25 percent of one-year-olds in Shelby County exhibited problem behaviors related to a lack of emotion regulation.

SOURCE: CANDLE Study (2009–2012) Parent report of social competence measured by BITSEA

Question:

Doesn't Shelby County already support social and emotional development?

Answer:

Yes and no. Today, Shelby County spends more time talking about child social and emotional development and its importance than in the past. But, schools, community organizations, and other local child service organizations have traditionally paid less attention to social and emotional development than cognitive outcomes and academic success.

Want to know more?

To learn more about the importance of social and emotional well-being, go to

http://www.urbanchildinstitute.org/articles/perceptions/kindergarten-readiness-is-more-than-academic

Why is it important to invest in social and emotional development?

One theory suggests that intervening with very young children at higher risk of social and emotional difficulties produces the largest gains in terms of skill development over time **(Figure 1.4)** [13]. Additionally, this theory suggests that this approach ends up costing communities or the larger society less money in the long run. In essence, pay now or pay more later. Unfortunately, a number of children struggle with at least one area of social and emotional development. These children and society may benefit from investments to set them on the best path forward. But we need to know what works, for whom, and under what circumstances, as well as where and how much to invest.

FIGURE 1.4

THE IMPACT OF INVESTING IN EARLY CHILDHOOD

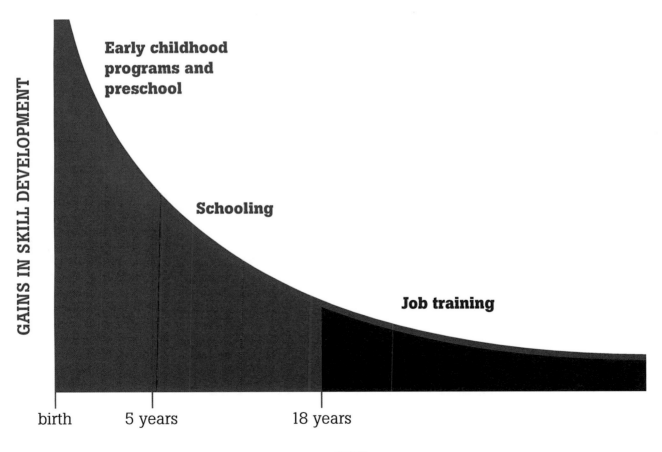

SOURCE: Adapted from http://heckmanequation.org/heckman-equation

How can this book help?

In the next chapters, *Off to a Good Start* explores the issue of social and emotional development in more detail and provides insights for how each of us can help.

There is no "one size fits all" approach. *Off to a Good Start* offers some quick tips to support child social and emotional development, but it is important to review the evidence when selecting a more comprehensive program or policy.

This book is designed to help improve understanding of the social and emotional development of children in Shelby County and help community members think about how they can make a difference.

To do this, the report pulls together data from both local sources of information and national sources. A list of these resources is available in **Appendix A.** The use of both local and national data highlights the knowledge available in Shelby County about social and emotional development, identifies differences and similarities between our local community and the overall United States, and emphasizes areas where additional information is needed to understand the local issues.

What is next in the book?

- Chapter Two provides a snapshot of the children living in Shelby County and their families, with attention to factors that influence social and emotional development.

- Chapter Three takes a closer look at factors in the home environment that could be addressed to support social and emotional development in young children.

- Chapter Four examines factors related to caregivers and child-care settings that could be addressed to support social and emotional development in younger children.

- Chapter Five summarizes the key findings from this book. This chapter also identifies action steps to promote and support healthy social and emotional development for the youngest residents of Shelby County.

Want to know more?

To learn more about the benefit of investing in early childhood, go to

http://heckmanequation.org/heckman-equation

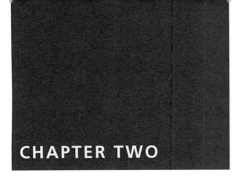

CHAPTER TWO

WHAT DO WE KNOW ABOUT THE
Children of
Shelby County?

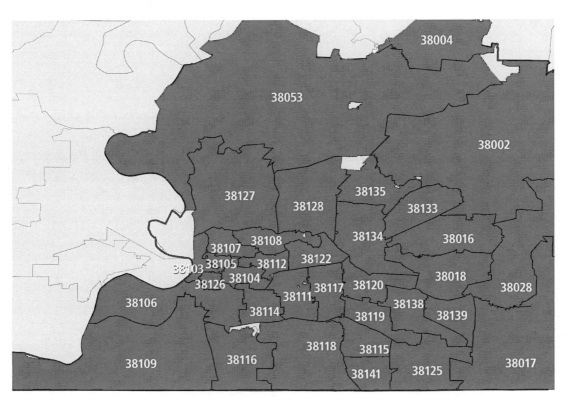

hapter One made the case that the first three years of a child's life are a time of incredible growth—physically, mentally, socially, and emotionally. This chapter drills down to focus on the children of Shelby County and their families, and on those factors that may influence the development of social and emotional competencies already described.

This chapter includes maps of Shelby County to show how these factors are spread out across the county. The map above provides information on the relative location of zip codes within Shelby County.

How many children live in Shelby County?

There are many young children in Shelby County. The 240,133 children in the county (under the age of 18) represent about one-quarter of the total population (26 percent), with a fairly even distribution across the age range **(Figure 2.1)**. Children under six (82,202) account for just under nine percent of the total population.

Within the City of Memphis, (163,322) children make up about one-quarter of the total population. Children under six years of age (59,662) account for 9 percent of the total Memphis population.

But where children live within Shelby County varies. The map on the next page **(Figure 2.2)** displays the distribution of children under the age of three by zip codes. Understanding the geographic distribution of children and the distribution of potential risk factors across Shelby County is useful for informing resource allocation decisions. The zip codes with the highest number of children cluster in three regions within the county, one to the south (zip codes 38115, 38116, 38118, 38109, 38111, 38125), one to the north (zip codes 38127, 38128), and one to the east (38018, 38016, 38134).

FIGURE 2.1

AGE

Shelby County children under the age of 18 years old

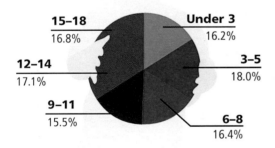

15–18 16.8%	**Under 3** 16.2%
12–14 17.1%	**3–5** 18.0%
9–11 15.5%	**6–8** 16.4%

The age distribution of children within Shelby County is similar to that of the state and nation. About 16 percent of children (38,975) are under three years of age. Slightly more (43,227, or 18.0 percent) are between the ages of three and five.

SOURCE: U.S. Census Bureau, American Community Survey 1-Year Estimates 2013, Table B09001

FIGURE 2.2

WHERE THEY LIVE

Shelby County children under three years of age by zip code

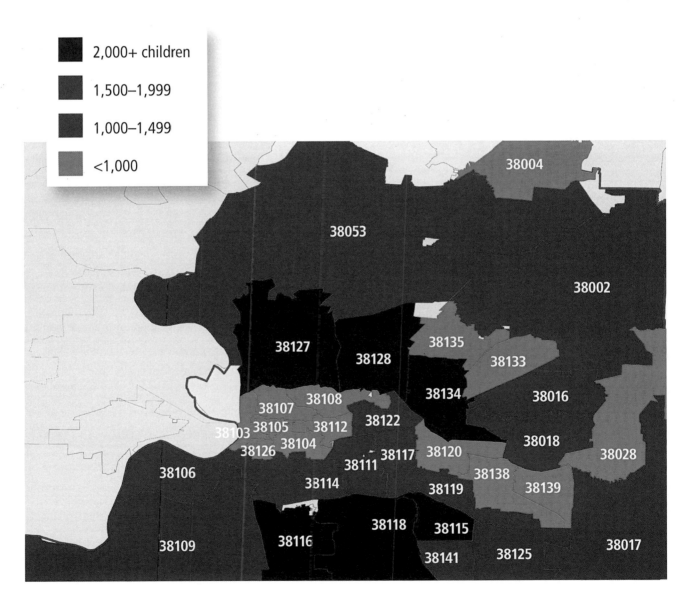

SOURCE: U.S. Census Bureau, American Community Survey 5-Year Estimates 2008–2012, Table B09001

What do we know about the health of newborn children?

In 2013, approximately 13,760 babies were born in Shelby County. While most are born healthy, many are born too early or too small. Infants born preterm (less than 37 weeks gestation) and at low birth weight (less than 2,500 grams or 5.5 pounds) are at greater risk for physical and developmental health problems, from poor lung functioning and language delays to infant death (death occurring in the first year of life).

Preterm birth can affect development.

In addition to physical problems, children born early tend to have more behavioral and social difficulties in the first few years of life [14].

Early birth affects the structure of the brain. When a baby is born early, the parts of the brain that receive, transfer, and store information have not had time to fully develop [15]. Why? At 34 weeks gestation, a baby's brain is only about 65 percent of the weight it would be if the baby were full-term (40 weeks). Preterm birth can also make child-parent bonding difficult because children born early often spend their first days, weeks, or months in the hospital, separated from their parents [15].

DATA FACTS:

- In 2013, 13 percent of babies born in Shelby County were preterm (1,790). While this percentage has remained relatively stable over time, it consistently hovers above the national figure of 12 percent.

- More black babies in Shelby County are born preterm (15 percent) than white babies (9 percent).

SOURCE: Tennessee Department of Health, Division of Policy, Planning and Assessment, Office of Health Statistics. Number of live births with number and percentage preterm, by race of mother and county of residence of mother, Tennessee, 2013

Low birth weight remains high in Shelby County.

Babies born early may have low birth weight. However, full-term babies can also be born with low birth weight if their mothers have high blood pressure; use drugs, alcohol, or tobacco; or do not gain enough weight during pregnancy. Children with low birth weight have poorer cognitive outcomes [16] and may also have behavioral problems, a harder time regulating their emotions, or be shy or withdrawn [17]. Nationally, about 3 percent of full-term babies were born with low birth weight in 2012.

When children have these difficulties, it can make parent-child bonding difficult (consider the hard-to-soothe child described in Chapter One). Low birth weight can also negatively influence how a child reacts to stress, making him or her more difficult to nurture.

Preterm babies	Full-term babies
- may have low birth weight - may have poorer cognitive outcomes - may have behavioral problems, be shy or withdrawn	- may still have low birth weight if mother has high blood pressure; uses drugs, alcohol, or tobacco; or does not gain enough weight during pregnancy - may still have low birth weight if born with a congenital or genetic problem

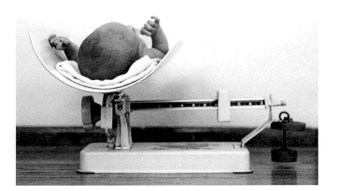

Want to know more?

To learn more about low birth weight, go to http://www.urbanchildinstitute.org/resources/infographics/low-birth-weight

DATA FACTS:

- In 2013, 1,611 babies (12 percent) in Shelby County were born with low birth weight. This is above the national average of 8 percent and the Healthy People 2020 goal of 8 percent.

- More black babies in Shelby County are born with low birth weight (15 percent) than white babies (7 percent).

SOURCE: Tennessee Department of Health, Division of Policy, Planning and Assessment, Office of Health Statistics. Number of live births with number and percent low birthweight, by race of mother and county of residence of mother, Tennessee, 2013

What do we know about the families of young children?

Family and experiences at home influence a child's social and emotional development.

Children's ethnic and cultural backgrounds influence their development.

Children's early life experiences are shaped, in part, by the backgrounds, cultures, languages, and beliefs of their families. By understanding these factors, we can ensure that support provided to the children and families of Shelby County is culturally and linguistically diverse, and is respectful of culture and beliefs.

Want to know more?

To learn more about culturally responsive parenting, go to

http://www.urbanchildinstitute.org/articles/ research-to-policy/practice/culturally-responsive-parenting

The distribution of children by race and ethnicity in Shelby County **(Figure 2.3)** is different than the United States overall. Nationwide, about 68 percent are white, about 14 percent are black, and 5 percent are Asian, with the remaining 14 percent reporting another race, or two or more races.

FIGURE 2.3

RACE OF CHILDREN UNDER 18

Shelby County families percentage by race/ethnicity

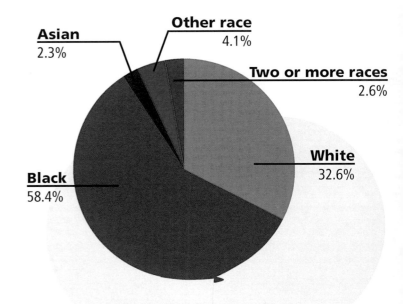

Asian 2.3%

Other race 4.1%

Two or more races 2.6%

White 32.6%

Black 58.4%

SOURCE: U.S. Census Bureau, American Community Survey 1-Year Estimates 2013, Table B01001A--I

FIGURE 2.4

LANGUAGE SPOKEN AT HOME

Percentage of people who speak another language at home, by zip code

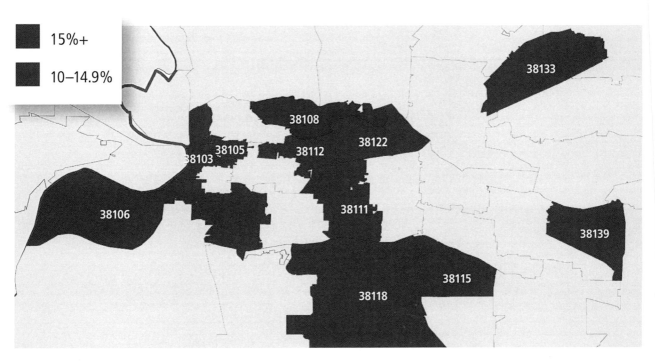

■ 15%+

■ 10–14.9%

SOURCE: U.S. Census Bureau, American Community Survey 5-Year Estimates 2008–2012, Table B16004

By ethnicity, about 9 percent of children in Shelby County and 10.9 percent in Memphis are Hispanic. Further, about 9 percent of individuals over age five speak another language in their home **(Figure 2.4).**

SOURCE: U.S. Census Bureau, American Community Survey 1-Year Estimates 2013, Table B010011

Poverty affects social and emotional development.

Children are one of the poorest groups in the United States [17]. Poverty can affect a child's development in different ways [17, 18]. Parents without stable and adequate incomes are less able to provide their children with stimulating environments, including books, educational toys, and enriching activities [19, 20]. Poverty is associated with other factors that negatively affect children's development. These factors might include unsafe environments, reduced access to healthy foods, and low-quality child care [21]. Poverty can also influence the social and emotional development of children by increasing stress and strain

FIGURE 2.5

WHERE THE POOR LIVE

Shelby County children under six living in poverty

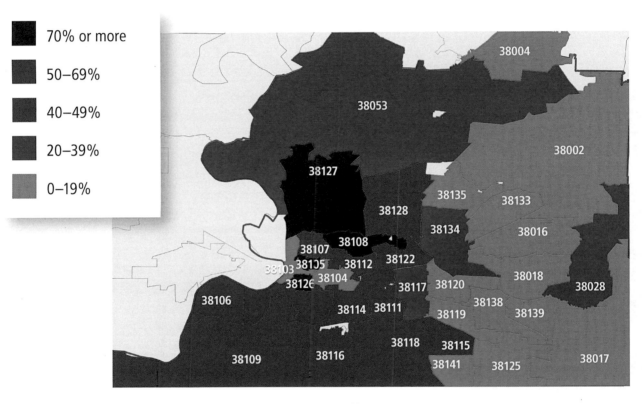

70% or more

50–69%

40–49%

20–39%

0–19%

SOURCE: U.S. Census Bureau, American Community Survey 5-Year Estimates 2008–2012, Table B17024

on families. This additional burden on caregivers makes it challenging to provide the nurturing parenting that children need to thrive in stressful environments.

The terms "poor" and "in poverty" are applied to families with annual incomes below the Federal Poverty Level (FPL) set by the U.S. Department of Health and Human Services. In 2013, the FPL for a family of four was $23,550.

In 2013, more than one-third (40 percent) of children under the age of six in Shelby County lived below

the FPL. In contrast, about a quarter (25 percent) of children under the age of six lived in poverty nationally in 2013. Areas of Shelby County to the north (38107, 38108, 38127, 38128) and south (38106, 38109, 38115, 38116, 38118, 38126) have the largest percentages of children under age six living in poverty, along with a few spots in the county's center (38105, 38111, 38112, 38114, 38122) **(Figure 2.5)**.

U.S. Census Bureau, American Community Survey 5-Year Estimates 2008–2012, Table B17024

FIGURE 2.6

CHILDREN LIVING IN POVERTY

Poverty among children under six in Shelby County

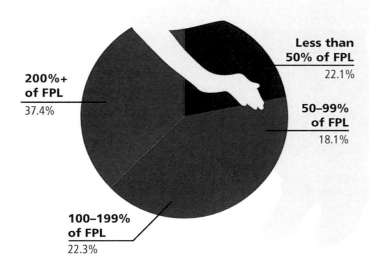

200%+ of FPL
37.4%

Less than 50% of FPL
22.1%

50–99% of FPL
18.1%

100–199% of FPL
22.3%

SOURCE: U.S. Census Bureau, American Community Survey 1-Year Estimates 2013, Table B17024

Not all poor children experience the same types of hardship, however. Some children live in extreme poverty (defined as an income that is less than 50 percent of the FPL) **(Figure 2.6)**. Other children live just above the FPL—but not by much—and face challenges similar to those living below the FPL. These children, in families with incomes between 100 and 199 percent of the FPL, are also quite poor, resulting in similar stresses and strains and fewer resources to create an enriching environment for the children.

The percentage of children in Shelby County living in poverty has increased over time **(Figure 2.7)**. More concerning is that this is driven largely by increases in the numbers of children living in extreme poverty, below 50 percent of the FPL.

Parental education also influences social and emotional development.

There are strong links between parent education and poverty. Parents with more years of schooling are more likely to get higher-paying and stable jobs. As a result, these parents may have more time and resources to provide a stimulating home environment for their children. For example, they are more likely to read more with their children and use a larger vocabulary when talking with them [22]. Mothers with higher levels of education also tend to display greater warmth and responsiveness to their children, like positive reactions when the child does something good or new, or hugs when the child is distressed, which contributes to fewer behavior and emotional problems [22].

FIGURE 2.7

PERCENTAGE OF CHILDREN LIVING IN POVERTY OVER TIME

Poverty among children under six in Shelby County

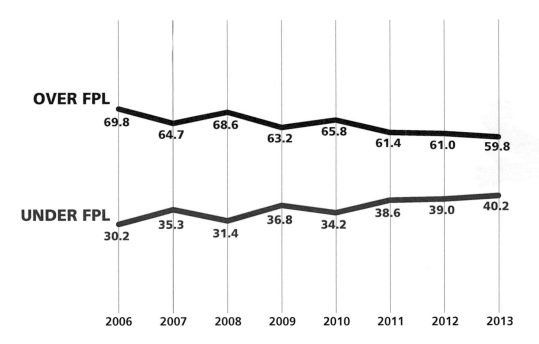

SOURCE: United States Census Bureau, American Community Survey, 1-Year Estimates, 2006–2013, Table B17024

HOW YOU CAN **help**

Offer your time, talent, or resources to a reputable nonprofit organization that offers services focused on improving the well-being of our community's young children and their families.

Consider prioritizing neighborhoods and communities of need when offering services that will benefit economically vulnerable families.

Encourage your religious congregation or social group to get involved in activities that support families with young children in disadvantaged neighborhoods.

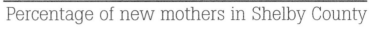

FIGURE 2.8

HOW MUCH MATERNAL EDUCATION

Percentage of new mothers in Shelby County

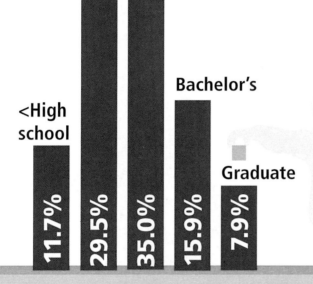

Some college

High school

Bachelor's

<High school

Graduate

11.7%

29.5%

35.0%

15.9%

7.9%

SOURCE: U.S. Census Bureau, American Community Survey 1-Year Estimates 2013, Table B13014

In contrast, children whose parents have less education may not benefit from these advantages and are less likely to meet some of the major milestones of social and emotional development outlined in Chapter One.

Within Shelby County, about 40 percent of women who gave birth within the past 12 months had less than or equal to a high school diploma. About a third had completed some college, and about 25 percent earned a bachelor's degree or higher **(Figure 2.8)**.

While this distribution is similar to the United States overall, within Shelby County there is significant variability as to where these mothers live. For instance, zip code 38108 has the highest concentration of new mothers with low education— more than half did not graduate from high school. As shown in **Figure 2.9,** there are a number of areas in Memphis where the percentage ranges from 20 percent to 49 percent.

FIGURE 2.9

PERCENTAGE OF MOTHERS WHO DID NOT GRADUATE FROM HIGH SCHOOL

Shelby County, by zip code

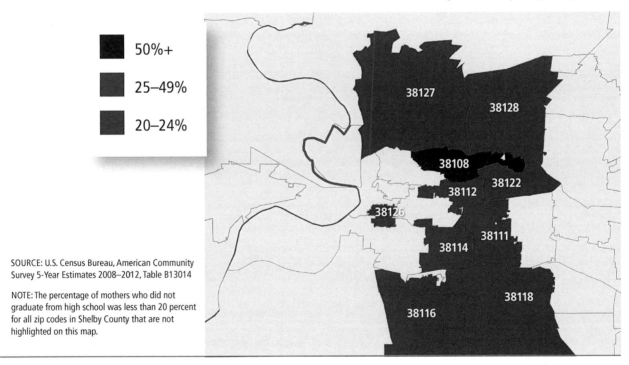

50%+

25–49%

20–24%

SOURCE: U.S. Census Bureau, American Community Survey 5-Year Estimates 2008–2012, Table B13014

NOTE: The percentage of mothers who did not graduate from high school was less than 20 percent for all zip codes in Shelby County that are not highlighted on this map.

HOW YOU CAN **help**

Consider serving as a tutor or mentor at schools or with literacy programs in Shelby County.

Emphasize to students, particularly young moms, how staying in school and graduating from high school is good for them and for their children.

Consider whether your organization could support new mothers pursuing educational opportunities.

CHILDREN LIVING IN SINGLE-PARENT HOUSEHOLDS

For children under 18, in Shelby County

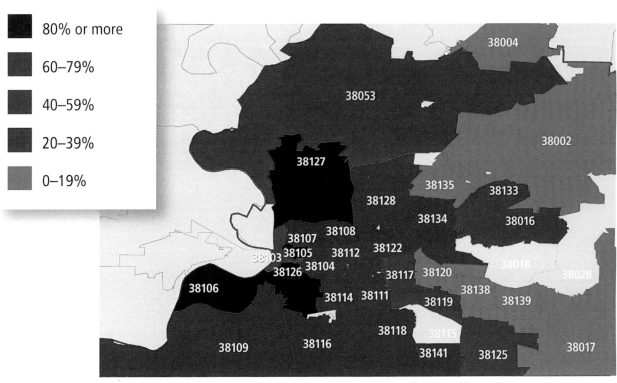

- 80% or more
- 60–79%
- 40–59%
- 20–39%
- 0–19%

SOURCE: United States Census Bureau, American Community Survey 5-Year Estimates, 2008–2012, Table B09002

More than half of children in Shelby County live in single-parent households.

In Shelby County, more than half (56 percent) of all children under six live in families headed by an unmarried parent **(Figure 2.10)**. Children who live in single-parent households tend to have greater behavioral and emotional problems than children who live in two-parent households. This risk is even higher for children who have lived with a single parent since birth [23, 24]. While many single parents are trying to do their best under difficult circumstances, many have fewer financial resources and may also have less support from friends or family to help out in times of need. This can increase parental stress, which may negatively affect parent-child interactions.

DATA FACT:

- In 2013, 49 percent of children in Shelby County under the age of 18 were living in single-parent households. This varied among zip codes and ranged from a low of 9 percent to a high of 96 percent. In zip code 38126, almost every child lived with only their mother or father.

SOURCE: U.S. Census Bureau, American Community Survey 1-Year Estimates 2013, Table B09002

FIGURE 2.11

LIVING ARRANGEMENT

For children under six, in Shelby County

Did you know?

▪ Just under 5% of children under the age of 18 have a grandparent living with them.

▪ In Shelby County, about 23,000 grandparents have one or more of their grandchildren living with them. About half are serving as the grandchild's primary caretaker or guardian.

Source: U.S. Census Bureau, American Community Survey 1-Year Estimates 2013, Table B10050

Both parents	Father only	Mother only
51.6%	**6.4%**	**42.2%**

SOURCE: U.S. Census Bureau, American Community Survey 1-Year Estimates 2013, Table B09002

Did you know?

▪ If a child is living with only one parent, it is more common for him/her to live with his/her mother, but many children live only with their father **(Figure 2.11)**.

▪ Areas where more than 10 percent of children live only with their father include: 38114 (19 percent), 38122 (13 percent), 38106 (12 percent), 38119 (12 percent), 38134 (12 percent), 38107 (11 percent), and 38053 (11 percent).

SOURCE: U.S. Census Bureau, American Community Survey 5-Year Estimates 2008–2012, Table B09002

HOW YOU CAN **help**

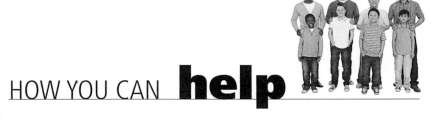

Create or support opportunities where single parents (including single fathers) can come together and support one another.

Strengthen fatherhood initiatives and support father involvement in child rearing.

Consider whether your program addresses the unique needs of single parents or grandparents raising their grandchildren, and whether these services could be expanded into new geographic areas of high need.

Children born to teen mothers are at increased risk for poor social and emotional outcomes.

Though the rates of teen pregnancy are declining, having a child early in life affects maternal education and job opportunities. Given that many teenage mothers will raise their children primarily on their own as single mothers, these challenges often result in fewer resources, added stress, and lowered social support for the mother. Teen parents are also less likely to receive timely prenatal care due to the unexpected nature of their pregnancies, which can have implications for their developing babies [25]. All of these factors have the potential to negatively affect children's social and emotional development.

DATA FACTS:

- Over the past few years, the teen birth rate has declined both in the state of Tennessee and in Shelby County, though it remains higher in Shelby County than in the state—and in the nation, where the birth rate was 29.4 in 2012 for girls between the ages of 15 and 19. (**Figure 2.12**).

- In 2012, 1,599 babies were born to mothers between the ages of 15 and 19 in Shelby County.

SOURCE: Tennessee Department of Health, 2002–2012

Conclusion

Many children in Shelby County live in poverty and have mothers who are single, young, and have less than a high school education. Research suggests that these factors, along with premature births and low birth weight, place children at a greater risk for social and emotional challenges. In the next two chapters, this book takes a closer look at factors in home and in child-care settings that may affect social and emotional development among young children. Each chapter also points to meaningful opportunities to improve the lives of children in our community.

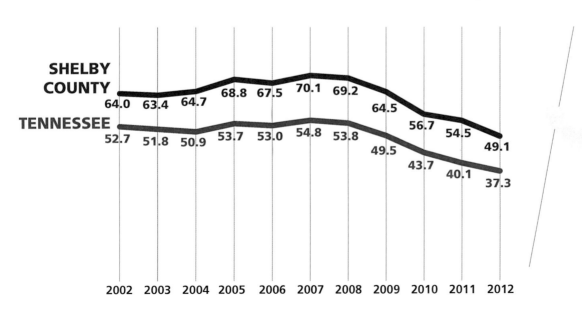

FIGURE 2.12

TEEN BIRTH RATE

Per 1,000 females age 15–19

SHELBY COUNTY: 64.0, 63.4, 64.7, 68.8, 67.5, 70.1, 69.2, 64.5, 56.7, 54.5, 49.1

TENNESSEE: 52.7, 51.8, 50.9, 53.7, 53.0, 54.8, 53.8, 49.5, 43.7, 40.1, 37.3

2002 2003 2004 2005 2006 2007 2008 2009 2010 2011 2012

Source: Tennessee Department of Health, Division of Policy, Planning and Assessment, Office of Health Statistics, 2002–2012

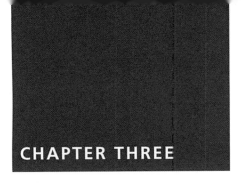

CHAPTER THREE

SOCIAL AND EMOTIONAL DEVELOPMENT
In the Home

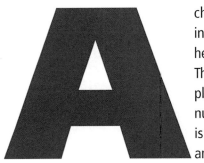child's home influences his or her development. The home is a safe place for play and nurturing, which is key for social and emotional development. The home is also where important interactions happen with parents, caregivers, friends, siblings, and others in the community.

This chapter focuses on the home environment and how positive interactions between parents and children can support healthy social and emotional development in early childhood. It also describes parental stress and parental mental health concerns in more detail. Both are significant influences on the social and emotional well-being of children, and help and support are available for both. This chapter concludes with a discussion of social support, which was touched on in Chapter Two.

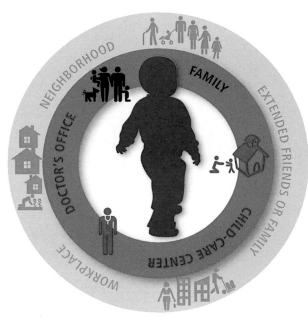

FIGURE 3.1

CIRCLES OF INFLUENCE

Did you know?

■ You can think of a child as being in the center of different circles of influence **(Figure 3.1).**

■ Family, day–care providers, peers, and religious institutions are most important for child development because the child spends the most time interacting directly with these groups.

■ The neighborhood where the child lives, a parent's workplace, and extended family or friends can influence the child indirectly through the impact on the parent or the environment.

SOURCE: Bronfenbrenner Ecological Systems Theory [26]

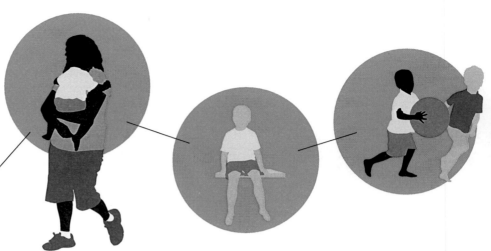

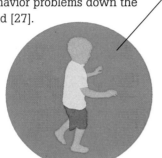

Did you know?

■ Parental warmth—touching, holding, comforting, rocking, singing, and talking calmly—can help children manage their emotional experience. This can contribute to the reduction of behavior problems down the road [27].

HOW YOU CAN
help

Encourage parents to provide warm, responsive, and sensitive support to their children and emphasize the importance of comforting, reading to, and talking and playing with children.

Consider supporting, developing, or expanding programs that will foster the development of positive parent-child interactions.

Model positive social and sharing behavior in your everyday interactions with children and parents.

Want to know more?

To learn more about positive parenting practices, go to

http://www.urbanchildinstitute.org/why-0-3/parenting

http://www.urbanchildinstitute.org/key-initiatives/touch-talk-read-play

http://www.rand.org/blog/2014/05/every-parent-can-be-a-better-parent.html

Parent-child interactions affect social and emotional development.

A child's relationship with a consistent, caring adult in the early years is associated with healthier behaviors, more positive peer interactions, increased ability to cope with stress, and better school performance later in life [17]. Babies who receive affection and nurturing from their parents have the best chance of healthy development.

Question:

What effect does warm, sensitive, and responsive parenting have on young children?

Answer:

It promotes feelings of safety and security, which provide children with the confidence to explore and engage with their surrounding environment. Children learn to trust that their parents will be there for them when they need something, when they are hurt, or when they have encountered something upsetting.

Figure 3.2 shows the proportion of parents who did not engage with their children in different activities that support positive parent-child interactions and social and emotional development of the child. Nationally, 15–20 percent of parents are not regularly engaging in these activities with their children.

SOURCE: National Household Education Surveys (NHES) Program Public-Use Data File, Early Childhood Program Participation, 2005. U.S. Department of Education National Center for Education Statistics

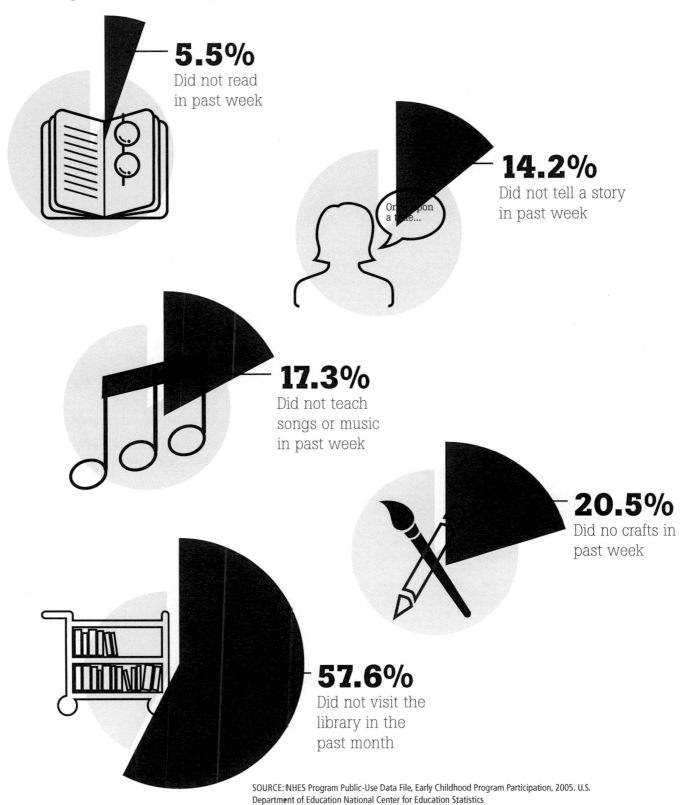

FIGURE 3.2

PARENT-CHILD INTERACTIONS

Percentage who do not engage regularly in these activities with their children

5.5%
Did not read
in past week

14.2%
Did not tell a story
in past week

Once upon a time...

17.3%
Did not teach
songs or music
in past week

20.5%
Did no crafts in
past week

57.6%
Did not visit the
library in the
past month

SOURCE: NHES Program Public-Use Data File, Early Childhood Program Participation, 2005. U.S.
Department of Education National Center for Education Statistics

NOTE: Age of child was three to five years, except for reading in past week, where ages were zero to five.

NOTES FROM THE FIELD

The University of Tennessee Le Bonheur Pediatric Clinic is implementing an evidence-based literacy program for young children called Reach Out and Read. This effort provides books at no cost to families at pediatric visits and encourages and demonstrates reading to children. Additionally, Shelby County Books from Birth—which is the local effort of Dolly Parton's Imagination Library program—distributes books at no cost monthly via mail to all children under five who are registered for the program.

Want to know more?

To learn more about local community resources for parents, go to

http://www.lebonheur.org/ulps/

http://www.reachoutandread.org

http://booksfrombirth.org

Parental stress may hinder the social and emotional development of children.

The developing brains of infants and toddlers are wired to expect responsive, warm, and sensitive interactions with parents and caregivers. But if that doesn't happen, children can suffer. Children in families experiencing hardship or poverty often witness stress, in the form of sadness and anger, from their parents and don't get the nurturing they need [28]. This can affect children's abilities to understand and read people's emotions [28]. Children as young as two can also experience sleep disturbances, become withdrawn, or display aggressive behaviors [29]. These and other negative behaviors can follow them into later childhood and adulthood.

DATA FACTS:

- In a national study of high-risk children in Early Head Start, approximately 28% of parents with children 12 months old report having high levels of parental stress [12].

- Using the same measure, approximately 15% of parents with children 12 months old in Shelby County report having high levels of parental stress.

- Mothers who are younger, single, have lower education levels, or are nonwhite are more likely to report having high levels of parental stress **(Figure 3.3).**

SOURCE: CANDLE Study (2009–2014) Parenting Stress Index (PSI) , percentage who met cutoff (>31) score for parental distress subscale

FIGURE 3.3

PARENTAL STRESS

Percentage of mothers in Shelby County who report high distress

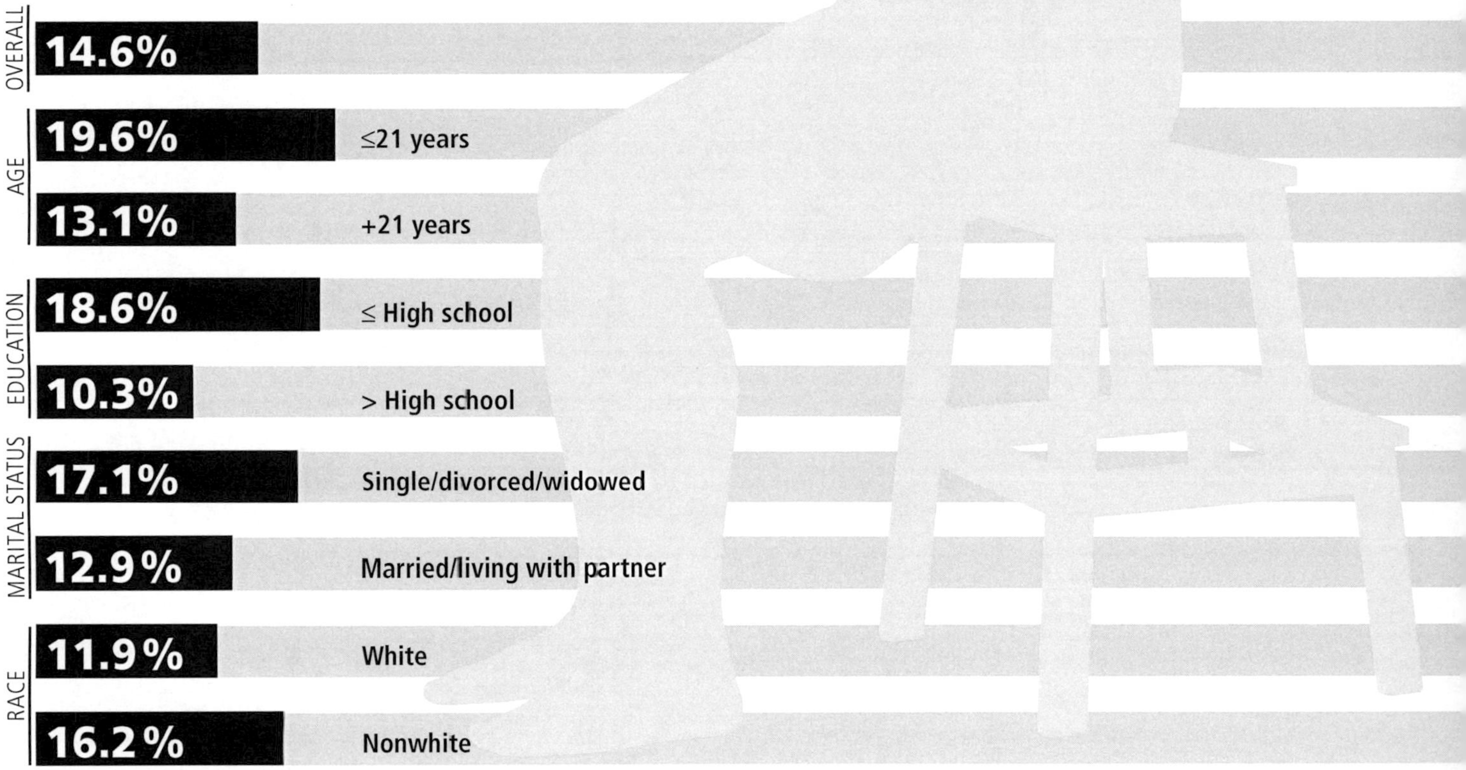

OVERALL	**14.6%**	
AGE	**19.6%**	≤21 years
	13.1%	+21 years
EDUCATION	**18.6%**	≤ High school
	10.3%	> High school
MARITAL STATUS	**17.1%**	Single/divorced/widowed
	12.9%	Married/living with partner
RACE	**11.9%**	White
	16.2%	Nonwhite

SOURCE: CANDLE Study (2009–2014) PSI, percentage who met cutoff (>31) score for parental distress subscale

Maternal or paternal depression may harm parent-child interactions.

Parental depression also poses a serious risk for healthy child development. If a parent has depression, he or she is less likely to provide rich, positive experiences that promote healthy social and emotional development. It can also compromise the quality of the parent–child relationship during critical years of development [30-34].

DATA FACTS:

- In the first year following childbirth, 7 percent to 13 percent of women experience depression [35].

- In a national study of high-risk children in Early Head Start, 17.6 percent of mothers of 12-month-olds experienced moderate to severe depression [36].

- In Shelby County, 5 percent of mothers of 12-month-olds reported symptoms indicative of depression, and nearly 10 percent of these mothers had possible depression (i.e., just under the threshold for depression). Mothers who were younger, single, had less education, or were nonwhite were more likely to be depressed **(Figure 3.4)**.

SOURCE: CANDLE Study (2009–2014) Edinburgh Postnatal Depression Scale (EPDS) at 12-month visit , percentage who met cutoff (10 or greater) for possible depression

Question:
How do you know if someone is depressed?

Answer:
Only a mental health professional can diagnose depression. But there are short tests that assess depressive symptoms. Individuals with more symptoms or who show symptoms for a longer period of time may be depressed and should see a mental health professional for help. But even without a clinical diagnosis, depressive symptoms can affect a parent and how that parent interacts with his or her child. So, it's important to support all parents who show signs of distress and mental health concerns.

HOW YOU CAN
help

If someone you know seems sad or withdrawn for a long period of time, and it is affecting his or her work or home life, encourage him or her to seek help from a professional.

Provide training or resources to parents and community members about how to combat stress and address mental health concerns.

Educate parents about the link between their emotional and mental health and their child's development and well-being.

Want to know more?

To learn more about maternal depression, go to

http://www.urbanchildinstitute.org/articles/perceptions/a-tale-of-two-children-part-5

http://www.rand.org/pubs/research_reports/RR404.html

Did you know?

■ Maternal anxiety and depression have been linked to a range of behavioral disorders in children in early life, including oppositional defiant disorder, attention deficit hyperactivity disorder, and conduct disorders [37, 38].

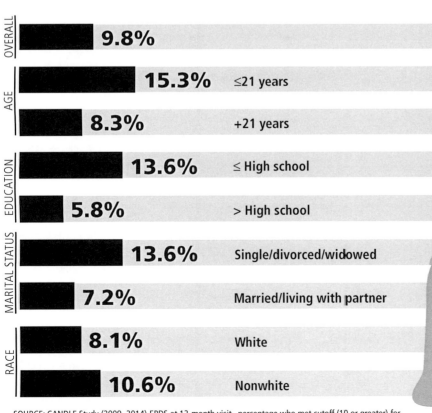

FIGURE 3.4

POSSIBLE DEPRESSION

Percentage of mothers in Shelby County with signs of depression

OVERALL
- 9.8%

AGE
- 15.3% ≤21 years
- 8.3% +21 years

EDUCATION
- 13.6% ≤ High school
- 5.8% > High school

MARITAL STATUS
- 13.6% Single/divorced/widowed
- 7.2% Married/living with partner

RACE
- 8.1% White
- 10.6% Nonwhite

SOURCE: CANDLE Study (2009–2014) EPDS at 12-month visit , percentage who met cutoff (10 or greater) for possible depression

Did you know?

■ Social support can be provided in many forms. It can include money, resources, companionship, or providing assistance with tasks such as child care or running errands [39].

HOW YOU CAN
help

Provide or support opportunities to grow and strengthen the social networks of mothers/parents and young families.

Help parents access high-quality child care, which may provide respite and lower maternal stress while expanding the parents support network.

Social support can help both parents and children.

It is important to have people you can count on for support, particularly when dealing with stress. Social support can reduce the emotional distress of the parent, and help improve the quality of parent-child relationships.

When support and encouragement is given to those caring for a child, adults are better able to be responsive and nurturing parents. Social support—both from trusted medical professionals and from less formal networks, such as friends, family, and a faith community—help reduce the stress that comes with raising a child.

Through providing parents with increased opportunities to complete school or job-training, or connecting them with local resources to address their own health, providers can utilize a more holistic approach to strengthen the family's well-being by addressing parents' needs, thus enhancing parent-child interaction, and in turn, children's development.

Conclusion

The development of social and emotional skills depends heavily on the experiences that children have in their home. Children can thrive with regular, positive, parent-child interactions. While parental stress and mental health concerns can jeopardize these interactions, mental health treatment and general social support of parents can alleviate some of the stress and strain of raising a child. This, in turn, will enable parents to focus more on their child and provide a warm, nurturing environment in their home.

CHAPTER FOUR

SOCIAL AND EMOTIONAL DEVELOPMENT
In Child-Care Settings

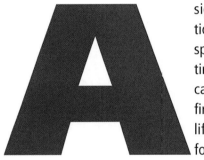

significant proportion of children spend at least some time in nonparental care during their first five years of life. This chapter focuses on aspects of nonparental care that shape the development of social and emotional competencies in young children **(Figure 4.1)**.

Similar to parent-child interactions, interactions that children have with nonparental caregivers can play an important role in promoting child development. This may be driven by the education level and training of the provider, as well as the overall quality of the nonparental care. The types of child care, including center-based, family child-care homes, relative care, or care in the home by a nonrelative—differ in their level of formality, the way they are set up, and the qualifications of the caregivers. This suggests that there may be unique needs for each setting to ensure that all children in Shelby County are receiving care in a way that maximizes their social and emotional development.

We focus much of the discussion in this chapter on formal (typically licensed) child-care providers, including center-based and family child care home settings. However, these issues can also apply to informal settings.

FIGURE 4.1

CIRCLES OF INFLUENCE

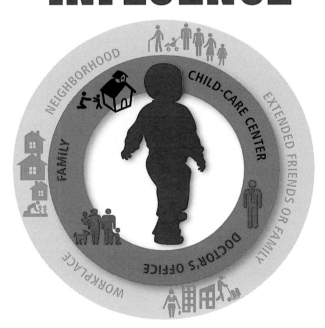

Formal child-care providers offer two main types of support important for children's social and emotional development [40, 41].

- Instructional support provides learning experiences or encourages skill development through interactions between a child and a child-care provider.

- Emotional support, defined by the warmth and sensitivity provided to the child, encourages the development of social and emotional competencies through responsive and supportive interactions [40, 42].

DATA FACTS:

- Nationally, only 13 percent of preschool teachers get high ratings on instructional support [43].

- Nationally, fewer than half of preschool teachers are rated as having a high level of emotional support [43].

Why are provider-child interactions important?

The interactions between children and their child-care providers contribute to the development of children's emerging social and emotional skills. Positive provider-child relationships in early childhood often include a high degree of warmth and closeness, a

Did you know?

■ Teacher interactions within preschool classrooms are stronger predictors of children's development than structural elements of the child-care setting (e.g., classroom design and space) [42], but these interactions are much harder to regulate.

minimal amount of conflict, and can occur when the child is able to share the provider with other children in the group setting [42-45].

Children who are in high-quality formal child care have:

- Increased social skills at the end of the preschool year [42]

- Improved academic school readiness [43]

- Less problem behavior at school entry and at the beginning of high school [42, 46]

- Better academic outcomes, which persist from school entry to the end of high school [46].

Question:

How can child-care providers improve their interactions with children?

Answer:

They can respond to children's developmental needs in ways that encourage them to try activities independently, while also providing them with guidance and help as needed. Through reassuring children they are safe, comforting them when they are upset, and making sure their basic needs are met, child-care providers give the emotional support that young children need to receive to develop trust in the child-care provider and other adults.

Question:

How can we improve the quality of interactions between child-care providers and children?

Answer:

One of the most promising avenues to support high-quality provider-child interactions is through professional development, typically for licensed providers. This includes training on positive interactions, behavior management, strategies for implement-

Want to know more?

To learn more about the importance of child care, go to

http://www.urbanchildinstitute.org/why-0-3/child-care

http://www.rand.org/blog/2013/04/give-poor-kids-a-chance-with-early-education.html

http://www.rand.org/blog/2013/02/rand-researchers-discuss-early-childhood-development.html

ing best practices, and the influence of responsive, sensitive caregiving on children's development [47]. A number of state initiatives, like the Quality Rating and Improvement Systems (QRIS), provide guidelines and a set of standards for centers and family child-care providers with the goal of improving the quality of care provided to children. Tennessee has its own QRIS—the Star-Quality Child Care program. Information on this program is described in the section titled "What Do We Know About Child Care Quality in Shelby County?"

Where do children spend their time?

Many children spend a significant amount of time in the care of someone other than their parents or guardians. Nationally, about 60 percent of children ages five and under who are not yet enrolled in school are in some form of nonparental child care on a weekly basis [48, 49] **(Figure 4.2).**

NOTES FROM THE FIELD

Tennessee is a partner state of the Center on the Social and Emotional Foundation for Early Learning (CSEFEL). CSEFEL is a national resource center for the dissemination of research and evidence-based practice. In Memphis and Shelby County, there is a growing awareness of the need for child-care providers to be trained more intentionally on the social and emotional development of children. Memphis community service providers recently used funds from a federal grant to employ experts in the CSEFEL model to train child-care providers in Shelby County on best practices in the healthy social and emotional development of children.

FIGURE 4.2

WHERE DO CHILDREN SPEND THEIR TIME?

Percentage of children birth through five, nationally

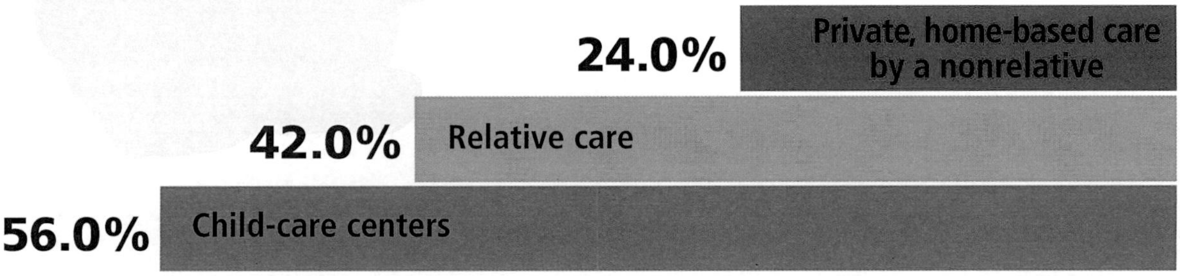

24.0% Private, home-based care by a nonrelative

42.0% Relative care

56.0% Child-care centers

SOURCE: Mamedova, S., and J. Redford, Early childhood program participation, from the National Household Education Surveys Program of 2012 (NCES 2013-029). National Center for Education Statistics, Institute of Education Sciences, U.S. Department of Education, Washington, D.C., 2013

Note: Categories are not mutually exclusive

FIGURE 4.3

WHO RECEIVES REGULAR NONPARENTAL CARE

Percentage of children, by age

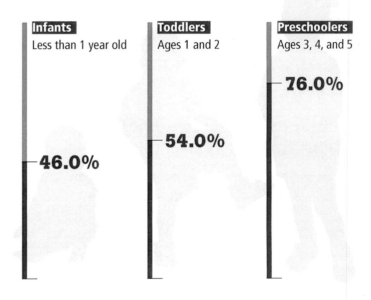

Infants
Less than 1 year old

Toddlers
Ages 1 and 2

Preschoolers
Ages 3, 4, and 5

76.0%

54.0%

46.0%

SOURCE: Table 1 from Mamedova and Redford (2013) [49]

FIGURE 4.4

WHO PROVIDES THE CARE

Where children spend their time when away from parents

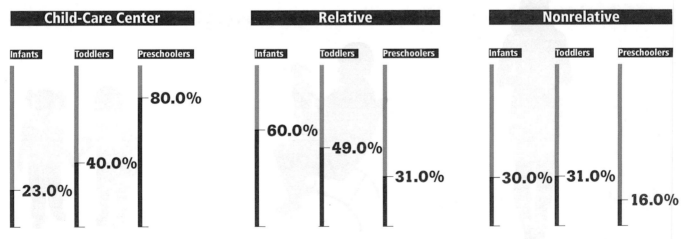

Child-Care Center

Infants | Toddlers | Preschoolers

80.0%

40.0%

23.0%

Relative

Infants | Toddlers | Preschoolers

60.0%

49.0%

31.0%

Nonrelative

Infants | Toddlers | Preschoolers

30.0% **31.0%**

16.0%

SOURCE: Table 1 from Mamedova and Redford (2013) [49]

The use of nonparental care and the type of non-parental care most typically used by parents varies by the age of the child **(Figure 4.3)**. Generally, use of care—and more specifically, use of center-based care—is greater for older children, ages 3 and 4 **(Figure 4.4)**. By then, most children are in center-based settings on a regular basis [49].

DATA FACT:

- Preschool-age children spend about 33 hours per week in child care [48].

What do we know about child-care quality in Shelby County?

Child-care quality is hard to measure in Shelby County because there is not a standard way to assess it. Currently, two programs are used to assess licensed child care quality above minimum licensing requirements: the Tennessee-initiated Star-Quality Child Care Program and National Association for the Education of Young Children (NAEYC) accreditation. Participation in either rating system is voluntary. Although measures of provider-child interactions are not assessed directly as part of the Star-Quality program, higher standards present in three-star providers or NAEYC-accredited centers may be more likely to foster positive provider-child interactions or promote positive social and emotional development. However, more work is needed to validate these rating scales with respect to social and emotional outcomes of children.

Star-Quality Rating System

The system **evaluates areas** such as professional development, developmental learning, parent/family involvement, program assessment, ratios and group size, and director qualifications.

It is **Tennessee-specific.**

Licensed centers and licensed family child-care homes are eligible.

The system has **star ratings of 0 through 3 that have increasingly more rigorous standards** for each rating level. A rating of zero stars indicates that a provider has met the minimum licensing requirements, but has not sought to strengthen the program beyond these requirements. In contrast, a three-star rating requires centers to have lower child-to-adult ratios for children ages one through three, additional hours of annual staff training that includes training in developmental learning standards, monthly written communication to parents, and an overall program assessment score equal to "good" or higher.

NAEYC Accreditation

This process **consists of ten standards that focus on children's learning and development** (e.g., positive relationships, curriculum content, assessments of children's progress), teacher qualifications, partnerships with families and the community, and program administration.

It **is national.**

It has standards that are highly regarded and **accepted as national standards** for centers.

It **requires centers to meet specific criteria** within each standard to become an accredited program.

TABLE 4.1

STAR RATING LEVELS

Among licensed providers participating in the Star–Quality program serving ages zero to five, by type of care

Shelby County	0 Stars	1 Star	2 Stars	3 Stars
All providers (N=527)	8%	1%	8%	82%
All centers (N=299)	6%	<1%	7%	87%
All family child-care homes (N=228)	10%	2%	10%	78%

SOURCE: Tennessee Child Care Management System for September 2014, provided by Child Care Resource and Referral (LeBonheur Community Health and Well Being Division)

NOTES FROM THE FIELD

There are ongoing efforts within our community to increase the quality of child care overall, and to improve the availability of high-quality, affordable care in neighborhoods where families have fewer resources. For example, one initiative called Ready, Set, Grow! has been working for more than ten years to provide resources to child-care centers in low-income areas with two or three stars to earn NAEYC accreditation. In addition, Le Bonheur Early Intervention and Development (LEAD) provides a variety of trainings and services to child-care providers to help improve quality of care.

DATA FACTS:

- About 67 percent of eligible Shelby County licensed child-care providers participate in the Star-Quality rating program. Of these, 87 percent of center-based providers have a three-star rating, and 78 percent of family child-care providers have a three-star rating. **Table 4.1** shows the distribution of the star ratings among providers who participated.

- In Shelby County, only about 7 percent of all licensed centers are accredited by NAEYC.

SOURCES: Tennessee Child Care Management System for September 2014, provided by Child Care Resource and Referral (LeBonheur Community Health and Well Being Division); NAEYC Accredited Program Search, http://www.naeyc.org/academy/accreditation/search

Where are three-star providers located?

It is helpful to understand the geographic distribution of higher-quality licensed child care across the county to identify areas of need and potential models of success. While this is difficult to assess due to the voluntary nature of the quality rating systems, we can get a glimpse into this by looking at child-care providers who participated in the Star-Quality rating system. The map in **Figure 4.5** shows the proportion of child-care slots in each zip code that are in three-star providers. This map does not include child-care

FIGURE 4.5

THREE-STAR CHILD-CARE PROVIDERS

Percentage of child-care slots with a three-star rating in Shelby County among child-care providers that participated in the Star-Quality rating system, by zip code

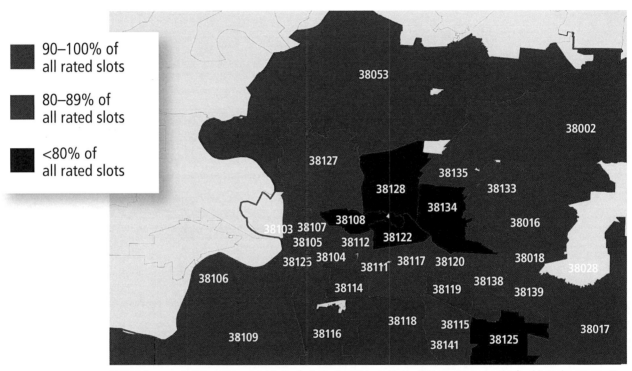

- 90–100% of all rated slots
- 80–89% of all rated slots
- <80% of all rated slots

SOURCE: Tennessee Child Care Management System for September 2014, provided by Child Care Resource and Referral (LeBonheur Community Health and Well Being Division); Capacity numbers provided through Department of Human Services Child-Care Providers Zip Code List—Shelby County (http://www.tn.gov/accweb/faces/stateMapPage.jsp)

NOTE: No providers in 38028 currently participate in the rating system.

Want to know more?

To learn more about improving access to and the quality of early child care, go to

http://www.memphis.edu/icl/rsg/

http://www.lebonheur.org/kids-health-wellness/le-bonheur-in-the-community/le-bonheur-early-intervention-and-development/

http://www.naeyc.org

http://www.maeycmemphis.org

http://www.rand.org/pubs/research_briefs/RB9639.html

http://www.rand.org/capabilities/solutions/improving-access-to-early-childhood-education.html

providers that did not participate in the Star-Quality rating system, including centers that are NAEYC-accredited but do not have a Star-Quality rating. As a result, it provides a limited look at child-care quality in Shelby County. Zip codes with the lowest proportion of three-star child-care slots include 38122 (54 percent), 38125 (72 percent), 38134 (72 percent), 38108 (78 percent), and 38128 (79 percent).

Question:

Why do you map child-care slots as opposed to child-care providers?

Answer:

Because centers and family child-care homes vary in size, child-care slots are a better measure of how many children can be served. As a result, it provides a better understanding of the proportion of children in a community who may be receiving higher quality care.

Conclusion

Children spend a substantial part of their time in nonparental care both inside and outside the home. Because of this, it is important to understand the current state of provider-child interactions that promote social and emotional health. Though little data exist to examine this locally, two quality-rating systems provide some insight. However, these systems have limitations, as well. First, they are voluntary, meaning there is no centralized data to examine child-care quality across Shelby County. Second, the Tennessee Star-Quality program does not explicitly capture provider-child interactions, which we know to be important. Third, they are not used to assess quality of provider-child interactions in more informal settings. Finding ways to improve child-care quality—and our measurement of quality—will increase the number of children who have access to high-quality care in Shelby County.

HOW YOU CAN **help**

Ensure that the child-care providers in your center or family child-care home participate in quality training on developmental learning standards, including the social and emotional development of children, as part of their required training hours.

Encourage frequent communication between providers and parents to ensure that children's developmental needs are being effectively addressed.

Partner with child-care centers that are "feeders" for kindergarten classes so that children entering school are familiar with the school before their first day. This will also allow teachers to be prepared for the incoming children.

Partner with child-care providers to ensure that services received are coordinated and complementary.

Work with families to identify high-quality child-care providers for their young children. Review the Department of Human Services (DHS) child-care locator and the NAEYC website to find three-star and NAEYC-accredited providers in areas close to parents' homes or work. Encourage parents to schedule a visit with potential providers to examine provider-child interactions and the overall environment.

Emphasize the importance of developmentally appropriate child care in the state of Tennessee by specifying minimum standards for developmental learning and provider-child interactions.

Want to know more?

To locate a child care provider near you, go to

http://www.naeyc.org/families/search

http://www.tn.gov/accweb/faces/stateMapPage.jsp;
jsessionid=5EF1706DAD417EC59D1F9BACAD12B4DC

CHAPTER FIVE

HOW PEOPLE IN THE COMMUNITY
Can Get Involved

This book highlights factors known to affect children's social and emotional development. While it does not cover all factors, mostly due to data gaps, it was designed to provide information on key factors that may be addressed or strengthened within the Shelby County community. These include factors in the home and child-care environment.

It is the hope of The Urban Child Institute that every reader of this book will identify some way in which he or she can support the social and emotional development of children in Shelby County. Some may be compelled by a topic, such as high rates of parental stress (particularly among younger, single mothers), while others may be more driven to make a difference in a specific community. Regardless, each effort, no matter how small or large, can positively affect the children of our community.

Where can individuals and organizations focus their efforts?

For the past ten years, community service providers in Shelby County have been proactive in educating themselves on the science of early childhood brain development and taking action to improve the state of young children in our county. This book has drawn attention to several efforts in Shelby County that are ongoing (a more complete list of organizations working in this area can be found in **Appendix B**). While investments have certainly grown, they remain

FIGURE 5.1

AREAS OF HIGHER RISK

Young children at higher risk for poorer social and emotional outcomes

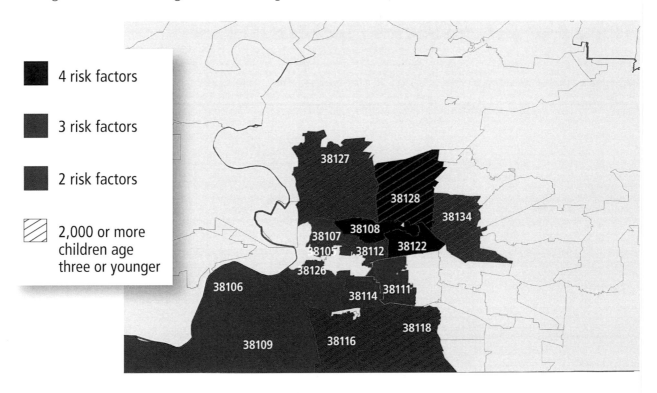

limited overall, and there are many opportunities to get involved.

While virtually every neighborhood within Shelby County would benefit from additional focus on the social and emotional development of its youngest citizens, there are several areas that are at higher risk for poor child outcomes. By examining communities where children face multiple risks to their social and emotional development, decisions about resource allocation and investments in the community can become data-driven, resulting in better outcomes and a higher return on investment.

The map above **(Figure 5.1)** provides information on the geographic regions at higher risk for poorer social and emotional outcomes among young children. It maps an index that includes several factors discussed earlier in the book:

- High proportion of zip code living in poverty (40 percent or more living below the FPL)

- Low maternal education (20 percent or more of mothers who did not graduate from high school)

- High proportion of single parents (40 percent or more of children who live with their single mother or single father)

- Lower-quality child care (fewer than 80 percent of child-care slots have a three-star rating)

The map also highlights those areas with a high concentration of young children (2,000 or more children ages three or younger). These areas may be worth particular attention.

As shown on the map, zip codes 38108, 38111, 38112, 38114, 38116, 38118, 38122, 38126, 38127, and 38128 have three or four risk factors. Of these,

FIGURE 5.2

43 | Off to a Good Start

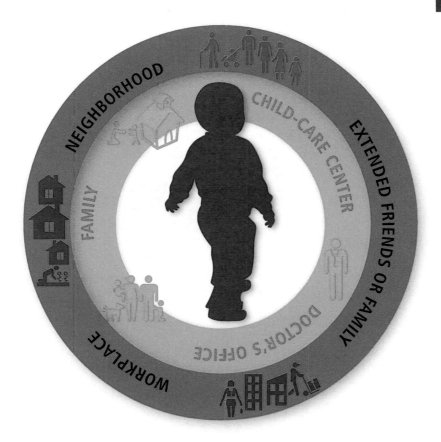

NEIGHBORHOOD

FAMILY

CHILD-CARE CENTER

EXTENDED FRIENDS OR FAMILY

DOCTOR'S OFFICE

WORKPLACE

38116, 38118, 38127, and 38128 also have the highest number of children, suggesting that these areas may be ripe for interventions or support and that such activities would reach a large number of young children with high need. It is important to note that the data presented in this map are illustrative. Other risk factors could be considered or the thresholds for "high risk" changed. As such, these data should not preclude investments in other zip codes or regions within Shelby County. The fact that a region is not highlighted on the map does not mean it wouldn't also benefit from investments. These data are intended to support and inform, not override, local knowledge and decisionmaking about resource allocation.

How can we leverage community assets?

As shown in the model of development that we have used throughout this book (Figure 5.2), child development does not exist in a vacuum. This book explored the home and child-care settings more specifically, but even these settings exist within a larger community structure.

For example, parents may be able to build social and emotional competencies of their children by taking them to programs and experiences within the community, such as story hour at the local library, or a nature walk at a local park, where children learn to interact with other children and adults in various settings. Child-care providers may take field trips to

FIGURE 5.3

COMMUNITY ASSETS

Areas with community assets such as libraries, zoos, museums, parks, playgrounds, and community gardens

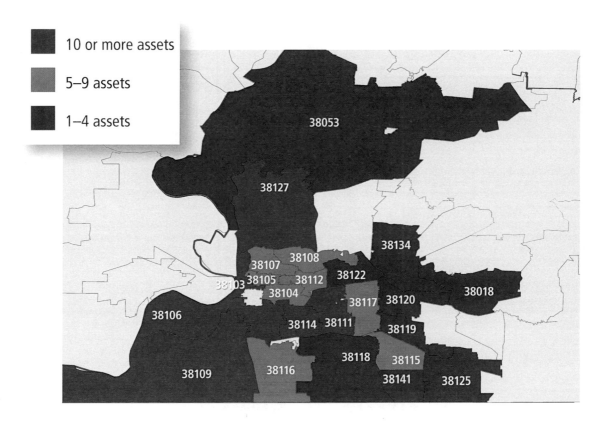

10 or more assets

5–9 assets

1–4 assets

the community garden or to the local fire station, again providing varied experiences for children and an opportunity to learn critical skills for how to interact in groups and behave in new settings. Such experiences do not have to be expensive; many are offered at no or low cost to the community. **Figure 5.3** maps out the location of several of these community assets: libraries, zoos, museums, parks, playgrounds, and community gardens. While there are likely other community assets not mapped, this is intended to provide a high-level snapshot of these assets and their relative location compared to the neighborhoods of opportunity noted above.

If you compare this map **(Figure 5.3)** to the map of risk factors in home and child-care settings **(Figure 5.1)** you may notice something surprising. Areas with the most high-risk children, in some instances, have many assets. Zip code 38127, for example, has 11 assets, while zip codes 38111 and 38114 each have ten. This is important to note, because communities may have important resources from which to build upon and there may be a community infrastructure that could be leveraged to support the social and emotional development of young children. Work may need to be done or investments made to improve the safety, quality, or quantity of offerings to young families (e.g., play groups at the park). It may also be that more efforts need to be made in connecting families to these community assets and resources, so they are aware of what is available.

Where is more information needed?

This book is just a start to summarize what we know about social and emotional well-being for children in Shelby County. While Appendix A provides a list of data sources that can provide additional information on social and emotional development, with the exception of the CANDLE data, little information is available at a local level to inform decisionmaking. We require more information to help us target resources and better meet the needs of young families. Here are some examples:

About the child:

Are there ways to track social and emotional development in children from birth to age five in Shelby County?

How does social and emotional development affect school readiness for children in Shelby County?

In the home:

What activities are parents and other caregivers doing to nurture child social and emotional development? How are fathers engaged?

What programs are best for Shelby County families to support the emotional readiness of children, and how might that differ by neighborhood or family background?

In the child-care setting:

How are children in kinship care (care of children by relatives) faring, and what supports are available to nurture social and emotional development?

What are child-care providers doing systematically to nurture social and emotional development? And what activities are best?

We need to better understand more about investments in supporting social and emotional development early in childhood that will have positive outcomes and cost savings down the road.

How to help

As noted throughout this book, there are numerous ways to help support the social and emotional development of young children in Shelby County. It is important to keep in mind that there is no "right way" to help; everyone in the community has different skills, resources, and time available. Providing an hour of child care for a mother who is highly stressed is just as important as expanding an evidence-based parent program into a new neighborhood. In this book, we focused on the home and child-care settings. Here are some ideas for each:

In the home or surrounding community:

Child-care providers can **work** with families to provide support and strengthen home-based strategies to cultivate child social and emotional skills.

Parents, other caregivers, and their supporters can **advocate** better programs that support social and emotional development. Determine what the needs are in the community, as well as what is working—and what is not.

Care for children. Provide a warm, nurturing environment and opportunities for them to explore, learn, and grow.

In the child-care setting:

Expand evidence-based practices that have demonstrated impact in supporting the social and emotional development of children.

Create new partnerships in the community. Are there organizations with whom you could partner that could support the development of social and emotional competencies of young children in your child care facility?

Train child-care providers, parents, and other adults responsible for the well-being of children. Given the importance of parent-child interactions and provider-child interactions for the development of social and emotional competencies, training and professional development opportunities should be made available that focus on these issues specifically.

Conclusion

Many children in Shelby County are at risk of not developing to their full potential. Many face multiple risks, including growing up in poverty and having younger mothers with less life experience and education. Raising a child in such an environment is exceedingly difficult for a parent and can result in higher stress, which in turn can affect the warmth and responsiveness of the parent toward the child. In addition, many children spend a significant amount of time in a child-care setting. Though many programs offer high-quality care, there are children spending time in programs that could be doing more to support their social and emotional development. As a community, we have a unique opportunity to consider these risks and the implications that they have for the children of Shelby County. Working together, we can help to strengthen these skills within our youngest children and set them up for lifelong success.

NOTES FROM THE FIELD

It's been said before that simple change can bring about tremendous results. It's often the slightest shift, the smallest adjustment, or the most unexpected turn that will lead to powerful transformation. With this in mind, The Urban Child Institute (UCI) will continue to lead a call to action, to focus our efforts and attention on the well-being of children in Shelby County during the critical ages of zero to three. Together, now, with the collaborative efforts of the RAND Corporation, UCI is dedicated to improving the lives of children and increasing the social capital of Memphis by using objective analysis to inform meaningful action that changes existing policies and programs. UCI is calling on you to join their efforts to make a change in the lives of our children and community.

UCI: http://www.urbanchildinstitute.org

RAND Corporation: http://www.rand.org

Want to know more?

To learn more about the promise of early childhood interventions, go to

http://www.rand.org/content/dam/rand/pubs/monographs/2005/RAND_MG341.pdf

DATA SOURCES RELEVANT TO
Social and Emotional Development

Data Source	Level of information available (National, state, county)	Description	Website
Conditions Affecting Neurocognitive Development and Learning in Early Childhood (CANDLE)*	County	An ongoing study of 1,500 Shelby County mothers and children starting from the second trimester and continuing through the child's fifth birthday, which provides information on the factors influencing young children's development.	http://candlestudy.com
Early Childhood Longitudinal Study*	National	This study includes three longitudinal cohorts that focus on child development, kindergarten readiness, and early experiences in school.	http://nces.ed.gov/ecls/
Early Head Start Family and Child Experiences (Baby FACES)*	National	Baby FACES is a longitudinal descriptive study of high-risk infants and offers a snapshot of Early Head Start programs, staff, families, and children.	http://www.acf.hhs.gov/ programs/opre/research/ project/early-head-start- family-and-child-experiences- study-baby-faces
Head Start Family and Child Experiences (FACES)	National	FACES is a descriptive longitudinal study of high-risk children and highlights the characteristics of Head Start programs, staff, children, and families. The experiences and outcomes of five cohorts of participating Head Start children have been tracked and described.	http://www.acf.hhs.gov/ programs/opre/research/ project/head-start-family- and-child-experiences- survey-faces
Head Start Program Information Report	National, state, and county	Data on staff qualifications, family and child demographics, and family use of additional services and resources.	http://eclkc.ohs.acf.hhs.gov/ hslc/data/pir

* Data source used in current report

Data Source	Level of information available (National, state, county)	Description	Website
Multi-State Study of PreK and Study of Statewide Early Education Programs	National	When combined, these two major studies of state-funded prekindergarten programs offer detailed information on teachers, children, and classrooms in 11 states.	http://fcd-us.org/ sites/default/files/ Prekindergartenin11States.pdf
National Household Education Surveys Program, Early Childhood Surveys*	National, regional	The School Readiness survey and Early Childhood Program Participation survey examine young children's use of nonparental care, early school experiences, and involvement in school readiness activities at home.	http://nces.ed.gov/nhes/ surveytopics_early.asp
National Study of the Incidence of Child Abuse and Neglect	National	This series of studies provide estimates of the incidence of child abuse and neglect, and examine this occurrence in relation to child and family characteristics.	https://www.childwelfare. gov/systemwide/statistics/nis. cfm
National Survey of Child and Adolescent Well-Being	National	This longitudinal survey examines the relationship between involvement with the child welfare system and child and family well-being.	http://www.acf.hhs.gov/ programs/opre/research/ project/national-survey-of-child-and-adolescent-well-being-nscaw
National Survey of Children's Health	National, state	The NSCH assesses children's physical and mental health, as well as their behavioral and social development.	http://childhealthdata.org/ learn/NSCH
National Survey of Children with Special Health Care Needs	National, state	Data from this survey provide information on the emotional, behavioral, and physical health of children with special health care needs.	http://childhealthdata.org/ learn/NS-CSHCN
National Survey of Early Care and Education	National	This survey assesses the nation's use of early child care and school-age care, with a particular focus regarding the experiences of low-income families.	http://www.acf.hhs.gov/ programs/opre/research/ project/national-survey-of-early-care-and-education-nsece-2010-2014
Panel Study of Income Dynamics (PSID)	National	This longitudinal study provides information on a wide array of data points, including child-rearing beliefs, child-care arrangements, and parent-child interactions.	http://simba.isr.umich.edu/ default.aspx
Study of Early Child Care and Youth Development*	National	This comprehensive longitudinal study is focused on child-care experiences, child-care characteristics, and children's developmental outcomes.	http://www.icpsr.umich. edu/icpsrweb/ICPSR/ studies/21940

* Data source used in current report

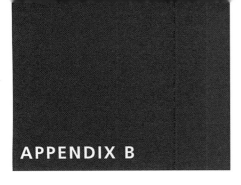

APPENDIX B

COMMUNITY ORGANIZATIONS SUPPORTING THE

Social and Emotional Development of Young Children

Community Organization	Target Population for Information and Services	Agency Description and Goals	Website
Agape Children and Family Services	Children, parents, community service providers	Dedicated to providing healthy homes for children and families through programs such as Families in Transition for homeless women and children and Powerlines Community Network, which serves families on site in the communities where they live.	http://www.agapemeanslove.org
Books from Birth	Children, caregivers, parents	Promotes kindergarten readiness and strengthens family bonds by providing age-appropriate books for all children from birth to age five.	http://booksfrombirth.org
Breastfeeding Coalition	Parents, community service and health providers	Promotes the importance of breastfeeding and provides supports to mothers who choose to breastfeed.	http://shelbycountybreastfeeding.org
Child Advocacy Center	Children, caregivers, families, parents	Serves children who are victims of sexual and severe physical abuse through prevention, education, and intervention.	https://www.memphiscac.org

Note. This list provides a sample of community organizations that support young children and is not intended to be exhaustive.

Community Organization	Target Population for Information and Services	Agency Description and Goals	Website
Early Success Coalition	Child care workers, community service providers, parents	Broad-based community collaborative to improve the lives of families with young children by improving birth outcomes, decreasing child abuse and neglect, and improving school readiness.	http://earlysuccesscoalition.com
Exchange Club	Children, caregivers, families, parents	Works to break the cycle of family violence and child abuse so that children do not grow up to become child abusers.	http://www.exchangeclub.net
Knowledge Quest	Children, families, parents	Designed to be the "tie" that binds connecting disparate sectors of the community—including businesses, churches, schools, and house-holds to improve the health of young people, families, and communities.	http://kqmemphis.org
Le Bonheur Center for Children and Parents	Children, families, parents	Provides prevention and early intervention services to children and families through home visitation programs such as the Nurse Family Partnership and Healthy Families—both evidence-based programs.	http://www.lebonheur.org/kids-health-wellness/le-bonheur-in-the-community/
Le Bonheur Early Intervention and Development (LEAD)	Children, child-care providers, families	Dedicated to working with children ages zero to three and their families to enhance developmental growth and independence in children and empower caregivers to become advocates.	http://www.lebonheur.org/kids-health-wellness/le-bonheur-in-the-community/le-bonheur-early-intervention-and-development/
Neighborhood Christian Center	Children, caregivers, families, parents	Builds stronger families and neighborhoods by provid-ing compassionate, Christ-centered ministries to those in need.	http://ncclife.org

Note. This list provides a sample of community organizations that support young children and is not intended to be exhaustive.

Community Organization	Target Population for Information and Services	Agency Description and Goals	Website
Porter Leath	Children, community service organizations, families	Provides needed social services to at-risk children and families in Memphis through a variety of initiatives and programs including Head Start and Early Head Start.	http://www.porterleath.org
Ready, Set, Grow! (RSG)	Children, business professionals, child-care providers	Mobilizes leaders in business, government, education, and the child-care community of Memphis around the common purpose that every young child in Shelby County cared for outside of his or her home receives the highest-quality care and education.	http://www.memphis.edu/icl/rsg/
Shelby County Office of Early Childhood and Youth	Children, caregivers, families, parents	Works to ensure children and youth have access to a coordinated, seamless network of both formal and informal resources in order to grow up, prosper, and contribute to a vibrant community life.	https://www.shelbycountytn.gov/index.aspx?NID=249
STRIVE/ Seeding Success Partnership	Business professionals, community service providers, policymakers	Focuses on improving reading and math success for children by building collaborations in the community and identifying data and measures to track success in these areas.	http://seeding-success.org
University of Tennessee Pediatric Clinic	Children, health care providers, parents	A partnership between The University of Tennessee Health Science Center (UTHSC) and Le Bonheur Children's Hospital. This pediatric practice is a teaching practice that serves thousands of children across Shelby County and includes the Reach Out and Read program—an evidence-based program to encourage reading early.	http://www.lebonheur.org/ulps/
The Urban Child Institute	Children, parents, child-care and community service providers	Focuses on promoting the healthy social and emotional development of children in the earliest years of life.	http://www.urbanchildinstitute.org

Note. This list provides a sample of community organizations that support young children and is not intended to be exhaustive.

Community Organization	Target Population for Information and Services	Agency Description and Goals	Website
Women's Foundation of Greater Memphis	Children, community service providers, women	Focuses on moving families living at or below the poverty level above the line toward economic security.	http://www.wfgm.org

Note. This list provides a sample of community organizations that support young children and is not intended to be exhaustive.

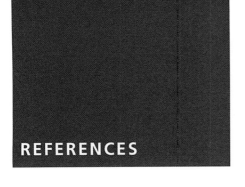

1. Gilmore, J.H., Lin, W., Prastawa, M.W., Looney, C.B., Sampath, Y., Vetsa, K., et al. (2007). Regional gray matter growth, sexual dimorphism, and cerebral asymmetry in the neonatal brain. *Journal of Neuroscience, 27*(6), 1255–1260.

2. Nowakowski, R.S. (2006). Stable neuron numbers from cradle to grave. *Proceedings of the National Academy of Sciences, 103*(33), 12219–12220.

3. Fox, S.E., Levitt, P., & Nelson, C.A., III. (2010). How the timing and quality of early experiences influence the development of brain architecture. *Child Development, 81*(1), 28–40.

4. National Scientific Council on the Developing Child. (2007). *The timing and quality of early experiences combine to shape brain architecture.* Working Paper No. 5.

5. Thomas, A., & Chess, S. (1977). *Temperament and development.* New York: Brunner/Mazel.

6. Putnam, S.P., Sanson, A.V., & Rothbart, M.K. (2002). Child temperament and parenting. *Handbook of Parenting, 1*, 255–277.

7. Ainsworth, M.D.S. (1979). Infant–mother attachment. *American Psychologist, 34*(10), p. 932.

8. Ainsworth, M.D.S., Blehar, M.C., Waters, E., & Wall, S. (1978). *Patterns of attachment: Assessed in the strange situation and at home.* Hillsdale, NJ: Erlbaum.

9. Sroufe, L.A. (2005). Attachment and development: A prospec- tive, longitudinal study from birth to adulthood. *Attachment & Human Development, 7*(4), pp. 349–367.

10. Sroufe, L. A., Egeland, B., Carlson, E., & Collins, W. A. (2005). Placing early attachment experiences in developmental context. In K. E. Grossmann, K. Grossmann, & E. Waters (Eds.), *The power of longitudinal attachment research: From infancy and childhood to adulthood.* New York: Guilford, pp. 48 – 70.

11. *Illinois Early Learning Project* website. (2014). Retrieved September 2014, from: http://illinoisearlylearning.org/

12. Vogel, C.A., Boller, K., Xue, Y., Blair, R., Aikens, N., Burwick, A., et al. (2011). *Learning as we go: A first snapshot of Early Head Start programs, staff, families, and children.* OPRE Report #2011-7, Washington, D.C.: Office of Planning, Research, and Evaluation, Administration for Children and Families, U.S. Department of Health and Human Services.

13. Heckman, J.J. (2006). Skill formation and the economics of investing in disadvantaged children. *Science, 312*(5782), 1900–1902

14. Morse, S.B., Zheng, H., Tang, Y., & Roth, J. (2009). Early school-age outcomes of late preterm infants. *Pediatrics, 123*(4), e622–e629.

15. Cepeda, I.L., Grunau, R.E., Weinberg, H., Herdman, A.T., Cheung, T., Liotti, M., et al. (2007). Magneto-encephalography study of brain dynamics in young children born extremely preterm. *International Congress Series, 1300,* 99–102.

16. Figlio, D.N., Guryan, J., Karbownik, K., & Roth, J. (2013). *The effects of poor neonatal health on children's cognitive development.* National Bureau of Economic Research.

17. Phillips, D.A. & Shonkoff, J.P. (2000). *From Neurons to Neighborhoods: The Science of Early Childhood Development.* National Academies Press.

18. Moore, K.A., Redd, Z., Burkhauser, M., Mbwana, K., & Collins, A. (2002) Children in poverty: Trends, consequences and policy options. *Child Trends, 2009-11.*

19. Eamon, M.K. (2000). Structural model of the effects of poverty on externalizing and internalizing behaviors of four-to five- year-old children. *Social Work Research, 24*(3), 143–154.

20. Yeung, W.J., Linver, M.R., & Brooks-Gunn, J. (2002). How money matters for young children's development: parental investment and family processes. *Child Development, 73*(6), 1861–1879.

21. Sklar, C. (2010). *Charting a new course for children in poverty: The reauthorization of the Temporary Assistance for Needy Families Program.* Washington D.C.: Zero to Three.

22. Davis-Kean, P.E. (2005). The influence of parent education and family income on child achievement: The indirect role of parental expectations and the home environment. *Journal of Family Psychology, 19*(2), 294.

23. Carlson, M.J. & Corcoran, M.E. (2001). Family structure and children's behavioral and cognitive outcomes. *Journal of Marriage and Family, 63*(3), 779–792.

24. McLanahan, S.S. (1995). *The consequences of nonmarital child-bearing for women, children, and society.* Report to Congress on out-of-wedlock childbearing. Washington, D.C.: U.S. Department of Health and Human Services.

25. Kaye, K. (2012). *Why it matters: Teen childbearing and infant health.* Washington, D.C.: The National Campaign to Prevent Teen and Unplanned Pregnancy.

26. Bronfenbrenner, U. (1979). *The ecology of human development: Experiments by nature and design.* Massachusetts: Harvard University Press.

27. Sabol, T.J., & Pianta, R.C. (2012). Patterns of school readiness forecast achievement and socioemotional development at the end of elementary school. *Child Development, 83*(1), 282–299.

28. Raikes, H.A. & Thompson, R.A. (2006). Family emotional climate, attachment security and young children's emotion knowledge in a high risk sample. *British Journal of Developmental Psychology, 24*(1), 89–104.

29. Rice, K.F. & Groves, B.M. (2005). *Hope and healing: A caregiver's guide to helping young children affected by trauma.* Washington, D.C.: Zero to Three.

30. Cummings, E.M., Schermerhorn, A.C., Keller, P.S., & Davies, P.T. (2008). Parental depressive symptoms, children's representations of family relationships, and child adjustment. *Social Development, 17*(2), 278–305.

31. Elgar, F.J., Mills, R.S.L., McGrath, P.J., Waschbusch, D.A., & Brownridge, D.A. (2007). Maternal and paternal depressive symptoms and child maladjustment: The mediating role of parental behavior. *Journal of Abnormal Child Psychology, 35*(6), 943–955.

32. Goodman, S.H., & Gotlib, I.H. (1999). Risk for psychopathology in the children of depressed mothers: A developmental model for understanding mechanisms of transmission. *Psychological Review, 106*(3), 458.

33. Lim, J., Wood, B.L., & Miller, B.D. (2008). Maternal depression and parenting in relation to child internalizing symptoms and asthma disease activity. *Journal of Family Psychology, 22*(2), 264.

34. Lovejoy, M.C., Graczyk, P.A., O'Hare, E., & Neuman, G. (2000). Maternal depression and parenting behavior: A meta-analytic review. *Clinical Psychology Review, 20*(5) 561–592.

35. Gaynes, B.N., Gavin, N., Meltzer-Brody, S., Lohr, K.N., Swinson, T., Gartlehner, G., & Miller, W.C. (2005). *Perinatal depression: Prevalence, screening accuracy, and screen- ing outcomes.* Evidence report/technology assessment (summary), 119, 1–8.

36. United States Department of Health and Human Services, Administration for Children and Families. (2011). *Early Head Start Research and Evaluation (EHSRE) Study, 1996-2010* Ann Arbor, Mich.: Interuniversity Consortium for Political and Social Research.

37. Shaw, D.S., Owens, E.B., Giovannelli, J., & Winslow, E.B. (2001). Infant and toddler pathways leading to early externalizing disorders. *Journal of the American Academy of Child & Adolescent Psychiatry, 40*(1), 36–43.

38. Latimer, K., Wilson, P., Kemp, J. Thompson, L., Sim, F., Gillberg, C., et al. (2012). Disruptive behaviour disorders: A systematic review of environmental antenatal and early years risk factors. *Child: Care, Health and Development, 38*(5), 611–628.

39. Manuel, J.I., Martinson, M.L., Bledsoe-Mansori, S.E., & Bellamy, J.L. (2012). The influence of stress and social support on depressive symptoms in mothers with young children. *Social Science & Medicine, 75*(11) 2013–2020.

40. La Paro, K.M., Pianta, R.C. , & Stuhlman, M. (2004). The classroom assessment scoring system: Findings from the prekindergarten year. *The Elementary School Journal, 104*(5), 409–426.

41. Pianta, R., Howes, C., Burchinal, M., Bryant, D., Clifford, R., Early, D., & Barbarin, O. (2005). Features of prekindergarten programs, classrooms, and teachers: Do they predict observed classroom quality and child-teacher interactions? *Applied Developmental Science, 9*(3), 144–159.

42. Mashburn, A.J., Pianta, R.C., Hamre, B.K., Downer, J.T., Barbarin, O.A., Bryant, D., et al. (2008). Measures of classroom quality in prekindergarten and children's development of academic, language, and social skills. *Child Development, 79*(3), 732–749.

43. Burchinal, M., Vandergrift, N., Pianta, R., & Mashburn, A. (2010). Threshold analysis of association between child care quality and child outcomes for low-income children in pre-kindergarten programs. *Early Childhood Research Quarterly, 25*(2), 166–176.

44. Howes, C., Burchinal, M., Pianta, R., Bryant, D., Early, D., Clifford, R., et al. (2008). Ready to learn? Children's pre-academic achievement in pre-kindergarten programs. *Early Childhood Research Quarterly, 23*(1), 27–50.

45. Sabol, T.J., & Pianta, R.C. (2012). Recent trends in research on teacher-child relationships. *Attachment & Human Development, 14*(3), 213–231.

46. Vandell, D.L., Belsky, J., Burchinal, M., Vandergrift, N., & Steinberg, L. (2010). Do effects of early child care extend to age 15 years? Results from the NICHD study of ear- ly child care and youth development. *Child Development, 81*(3), 737–756.

47. Hamre, B.K, (2012). A Course on Effective Teacher-Child Interactions Effects on Teacher Beliefs, Knowledge, and Observed Practice. *American Education Research Journal, 49*(1), 88–123.

48. Laughlin, L. (2011). *Who's Minding the Kids?: Child Care Arrangements.* U.S. Department of Commerce, Bureau of the Census.

49. Mamedova, S., & Redford, J. (2013). *Early childhood program participation, from the National Household Education Surveys Program of 2012 (NCES 2013-029).* Washington, D.C.: National Center for Education Statistics, Institute of Education Sciences, U.S. Department of Education.